Essentials of

Immunization

with Frequently Asked Questions and Answers

Essentials of
Immunization
with Frequently Asked Questions and Answers

Bhola Nath
MBBS, MD, DNB, MIPHA, DFM
Associate Professor
Department of Community Medicine
VCSG Government Institute of Medical Sciences and Research
Srinagar, Uttarakhand

Editor-in-Chief
Journal of Forensic and Community Medicine
Journal of Preventive Medicine and Holistic Health

Ranjeeta Kumari
MBBS, MD, DNB, MIPHA
Assistant Professor
Department of Community and Family Medicine
All India Institute of Medical Sciences
Rishikesh, Uttarakhand

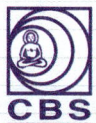

CBS Publishers & Distributors Pvt Ltd

New Delhi • Bengaluru • Chennai • Kochi • Kolkata • Mumbai
Hyderabad • Nagpur • Patna • Pune • Vijayawada

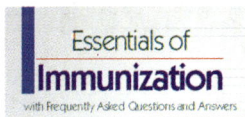

Essentials of
Immunization
with Frequently Asked Questions and Answers

ISBN: 978-81-239-2897-5

Copyright © Authors and Publisher

First Edition: 2016

Published by Satish Kumar Jain and produced by Varun Jain for

CBS Publishers & Distributors Pvt Ltd

4819/XI Prahlad Street, 24 Ansari Road, Daryaganj, New Delhi 110 002, India.

Ph: 23289259, 23266861, 23266867   Website: www.cbspd.com

Fax: 011-23243014   e-mail: delhi@cbspd.com; cbspubs@airtelmail.in.

Corporate Office : 204 FIE, Industrial Area, Patapparganj, Delhi 110092

Ph: 4934 4934   Fax: 4934 4935   e-mail: publishing@cbspd.com; publicity@cbspd.com

Branches

- **Bengaluru:** Seema House 2975, 17th Cross, K.R. Road,
  Banasankari 2nd Stage, Bengaluru 560 070, Karnataka
  Ph: +91-80-26771678/79   Fax: +91-80-26771680   e-mail: bangalore@cbspd.com
- **Chennai:** 7, Subbaraya Street, Shenoy Nagar, Chennai 600 030, Tamil Nadu
  Ph: +91-44-26680620, 26681266   Fax: +91-44-42032115   e-mail: chennai@cbspd.com
- **Kochi:** Ashana House, No. 39/1904, AM Thomas Road, Valanjambalam, Ernakulam 682 018,
  Kochi, Kerala
  Ph: +91-484-4059061-65   Fax: +91-484-4059065   e-mail: kochi@cbspd.com
- **Kolkata:** 6/B, Ground Floor, Rameswar Shaw Road, Kolkata-700 014, West Bengal
  Ph: +91-33-22891126, 22891127, 22891128   e-mail: kolkata@cbspd.com
- **Mumbai:** 83-C, Dr E Moses Road, Worli, Mumbai-400018, Maharashtra
  Ph: +91-22-24902340/41   Fax: +91-22-24902342   e-mail: mumbai@cbspd.com

Representatives

- **Hyderabad**   0-9885175004   • **Nagpur**   0-9021734563
- **Patna**   0-9334159340   • **Pune**   0-9623451994
- **Vijayawada**   0-9000660880

Printed At : Goyal Offset Printers

to
our
dearest
Almighty God
for guiding us
in this endeavour

Preface

It is a matter of great pleasure for us to write the book entitled *Essentials of Immunization*. The idea to write this book was conceptualized during our junior residency in the Department of Community Medicine about ten years back when we used to teach immunization and also practise it in clinics as an essential part of curriculum and preventive services under community medicine specialty. This idea has incubated over a long period of time so that we could gain sufficient experience in this area and also collect experiences from others such as colleagues, students and other health care personnel involved in delivering this important preventive service.

While teaching undergraduate and postgraduate students over the years, we have observed that a lot of queries related to immunization exist. These queries are both theoretical as well as practical in nature. Immunization, being a key preventive intervention for almost all communicable diseases, is an essential part of undergraduate curriculum as well as postgraduate curriculum in community medicine, pediatrics as well as nursing and contributes a significant proportion in their theory and practical examinations. Apart from the examination point of view, immunization is also a very important preventive service offered to individuals, specially children, for protection against various deadly diseases. It is important to remember that diseases such as smallpox which were once deadly, could have been eradicated by this single intervention. In today's context also, immunization continues to make its contribution to the health of the people.

This book has been written in a very simple and systematic manner so that the students can derive maximum benefit from the contents of the book. The book initially describes about the general principles of immunization, safe injection practices, adverse events following immunization and then moves onto describing individual vaccines in a comprehensive manner. The core strength of the book is that each chapter is followed by frequently asked questions related to a particular vaccine. These questions are frequently encountered by the students as well as health professionals during their examination and later during delivery of health care services. We hope that this book will be valuable for everyone involved in immunization, especially the students who are learning the basic concepts of immunization, as well as those preparing for their postgraduate medical entrance examinations.

Bhola Nath
Ranjeeta Kumari

Acknowledgments

First of all, we would like to thank the Almighty whose grace, blessings and guidance are indescribable and countless. The whole book specially the FAQs part of the book has been prepared after a lot of efforts and enquiries made from pediatricians, public health professionals and medical students. Over the course of an academic carrier we have had the pleasure of meeting and working with many faculty members and individuals who have enriched our knowledge in immunization. Our sincere thanks to medical students, whose queries have made us capable of thinking, rethinking and searching answers to the queries and finally paved the path of penning them down in the shape of this book. We hope that our other colleagues, too many to name, who have been such a pleasure to work with over the years of our academic career will accept our thanks. Our heartfelt thanks to Mr Brij Bhushan Bhasin, our friend, philosopher and guide, who ably and enthusiastically motivated us to turn our ideas into a readable form. We would also like to thank to our senior teachers whose constant support was always with us, especially Prof JV Singh who was our guide and mentor during postgraduation and had incited our interest in immunization by making us undertake our thesis on immunization. We would also like to thank Dr ND Vaswani and Dr Tanu Midha who were always ready to extend a helping hand whenever it was needed.

Finally, and most important of all, we wish to thank all the members of our "extended" family especially Mrs Kavita Vaswani and our kids Tuktuk, Happy and Pumpkin whose love and unending support has helped us in turning this dream into a reality.

Bhola Nath
Ranjeeta Kumari

Contents

Preface   *vii*

1. General Considerations about Vaccines   1

2. Safe Injection Practices   17

3. Adverse Events Following Immunization (AEFI)   21

4. Cold Chain   23

5. National Immunization Schedule   36

6. Planning an Immunization Session   43

7. BCG Vaccine   46

8. Dophtheria, Pertussis and Tetanus (DPT) Vaccine   50

9. Tetanus Vaccine   60

10. Measles Vaccine   67

11. Rubella Vaccine   73

12. Mumps Vaccine   75

13. Poliomyelitis Vaccine   77

14. Viral Hepatitis   86

15. Chickenpox Vaccine   93

16. Meningococcal Meningitis Vaccine   98

17. Influenza Virus Vaccine   102

18. Haemophilus Influenzae Type b (Hib) Vaccine   104

19. Pneumococcal Vaccine   107

20. Rotavirus Vaccine   110

21. Typhoid Vaccine   112

22. Cholera Vaccine   116

23. Rabies Vaccine   119

24. Japanese Encephalitis Vaccine   128

25. Vaccines for Yellow Fever, Leptospirosis, Kyasanur
Forest Disease, and Brucellosis   130

26. Plague Vaccine   132

27. Human Papillomavirus (HPV) Vaccine   134

Appendix
Comprehensive Table of Common Vaccines   137

Index   145

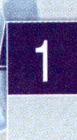

General Considerations about Vaccines

Immunization: It is a process of producing immunity in the host by active or passive methods.

Active immunization requires administration of "Antigen" (commonly known as vaccines), which can be in various forms such as killed/inactivated microorganisms, live attenuated micro-organisms, a part of the microorganism such as polysaccharide, a subunit, etc. The body responds to this antigen and develops antigen-specific humoral and cellular immunity after a variable period of time of administration of the antigen. However, the immunity that is developed, stays for long time. The cost of producing vaccines is less as compared to an immunoglobulin.

Passive immunization includes administration of preformed antibodies (commonly known as immunoglobulins) to the individual. Since the antibodies are preformed, the protection provided is immediate. But the process of preparing ready-made antibodies, similar to that of a ready-made dinner will be costly! Also, the duration of protection will be short lived. These immunoglobulins can be obtained from humans (homologous) or from animals (heterologous). Homologous immunoglobulin usually contain many different kinds of antibodies (polyclonal). When the antibody is produced from a single clone of B cells, it contains antibody to only one antigen or closely related groups of antigen (monoclonal antibody). The body accepts homologous antibodies better than heterologous antibodies, since heterologous antibodies are derived from another species. Therefore, the adverse reactions to homologous immunoglobulins are milder as compared to heterologous immunoglobulins.

Therefore, the two broad types of immunizing agents are as follows:

- Vaccines (for active immunity)
- Immunoglobulins (for passive immunity)

Vaccines are further classified into following different types based on their components and mechanism of production:

- Live attenuated vaccines
- Inactivated/killed vaccines
- Toxoids
- Combinations

Below are listed important points about each type of vaccines:

1. LIVE ATTENUATED VACCINES

These vaccines contain living microorganisms, which have been attenuated or weakened or modified to such an extent in a laboratory that they retain their potential to generate immune response in the body, but they are unable to cause a disease in a normal healthy individual. There is a "theoretical" and "rare" risk of the live microorganism mutating and developing into a virulent form to cause a disease. Therefore, live attenuated vaccines are contraindicated in individuals with compromised immunity due to various reasons such as diseases like cancers, HIV, etc. or physiological states such as pregnancy or in case of intake of certain medicines such as steroids and chemotherapeutic agents which might compromise the immune status of an individual. The storage conditions for these vaccines are stringent and the temperature during storage and transport has to be maintained strictly within the recommended limits. Live attenuated viral vaccines are easier to prepare as compared to live attenuated bacterial vaccines, due to the differences in their genetic constitution. They produce prolonged immunity usually with a single dose (exception: OPV, Rotavirus, since they are not fully taken up by the body due to losses that occur because of their route of administration, i.e. oral route).

Classification of live attenuated vaccines:

- *Bacterial* (Mnemonic: TBC)
  - **Typhoid** oral
  - **BCG**
  - **Cholera**

- *Viral* (Mnemonic: R²OMMIYO J (Rommiyo J))
  - **R**ubella
  - **R**otavirus
  - **O**ral polio
  - **M**umps
  - **M**easles
  - **I**nfluenza
  - **Y**ellow fever
  - **O**KA strain of chicken pox
  - **J**apanese encephalitis
- *Rickettsial:* Epidemic typhus

2. INACTIVATED/KILLED VACCINES

These vaccines contain killed or inactivated microorganisms. The inactivation is done through the application of heat, irradiation or chemicals like phenol or formalin etc. These micro-organisms, unlike those in live attenuated vaccines cannot replicate at all. Therefore, the immunity provided is usually short-lived and requires multiple doses. Since they are devoid of live micro-organisms, they can be given safely to people with compromised immunity, their storage conditions are not stringent, and the cost of production is less than live attenuated vaccines.

Classification of Inactivated Vaccines

- Inactivated vaccines (depending on the whole or part of microorganisms)
  1. Whole microorganisms
  2. Fraction/subunit (depending on the components)
     i. Protein
        a. Naked DNA vaccine
        b. Recombinant DNA vaccine
     ii. Polysaccharide (depending on the conjugation)
        a. Pure polysaccharide
        b. Conjugated polysaccharide

Inactivated vaccines can contain either whole microorganisms or a part of it **(fraction/subunit)**.

Fractional/subunit vaccines are refined vaccines and contain only a part of the bacteria/virus. Depending on the components of the vaccine, subunit vaccines can further be classified into *protein based* or *polysaccharide based* depending on the components of the microorganism that they contain. Since these vaccines have only specific immunogenic components of the bacteria, they are less likely to produce adverse reactions.

The polysaccharide based vaccines contain the polysaccharide wall of the bacteria. Polysaccharide coatings disguise a bacterium's antigens, therefore making them unrecognizable by the immature immune system of infants and younger children. The immune response to a **pure polysaccharide vaccine** is typically **T cell independent** and therefore, the infants are unable to produce consistent responses to these vaccines. Also, since IgM is the predominant antibody produced in response to most poly-saccharide vaccines, the repeat doses of a polysaccharide vaccine usually do not cause a booster effect.

To overcome these problems, the polysaccharides are linked to a protein or antigens that the infant's immune system can recognize. Such vaccines which contain polysaccharides chemically linked with a protein are known as **conjugate polysaccharide vaccines**. Conjugation changes the immune response from T cell independent to T cell dependent, thereby leading to increased immune response in infants and also booster effect from multiple doses.

Examples: Hib, pneumococcal and meningococcal.

Remember: In infants, conjugate polysaccharide vaccines should be given for optimum immune response, instead of a pure polysaccharide vaccine. The differences between pure poly-saccharide and conjugate vaccines are listed in Table 1.1.

DNA vaccines: When the subunit vaccines contain antigens in the form of genetic material of the microbes instead of the whole cell or the cell wall, etc. they are known as **DNA vaccines**. The DNA vaccines use the genetic materials that code for the immunogenic antigens as the component of the vaccine. DNA vaccines could be further classified into 2 types:

- Naked DNA vaccine
- Recombinant DNA vaccine.

The **naked DNA vaccines** consist of DNA that is administered directly into the body of the individual. When an attenuated virus or bacteria is used to introduce DNA of the microbe into the cells

Table 1.1: Differences between pure polysaccharide and conjugate vaccines

Characteristics	Pure poly-saccharide	Conjugate
T cell dependent immune response	No	Yes
Immune memory	No	Yes
Lack of hyporesponsiveness	No	Yes
Booster effect	No	Yes
Herd immunity	No	Yes
Reduction of carriage	No	Yes
Administration in infants	No	Yes
Duration of protection	Short	Long
Control of outbreak/epidemic	Yes	No

of the body similar to the process of a viral infection, the vaccine is known as a **recombinant DNA vaccine/recombinant vector vaccine,** in which the virus or the bacteria serve as vector for the microbial genetic material.

Inactivated vaccines can safely be administered to an individual with immunodeficient state. It requires multiple doses, the first dose is for priming the immune system and the subsequent doses produce the optimum levels of immune status. Usually, the humoral immunity is produced in response to inactivated vaccines and booster doses might be required to maintain optimum levels of immunity. The differences between the attenuated and killed/inactivated vaccines are listed in Table 1.2.

Remember: The main advantage of an inactivated vaccine is that it can be given to immunodeficient individuals.

3. TOXOIDS

They are made from bacteria that secrete toxins or harmful chemicals in the process of pathogenesis for causing illness. These toxins are inactivated by chemicals, etc. and used as "toxoids". The immune system is primed to fight against the natural toxin, when it receives the harmless toxin in the form of toxoid, e.g. diphtheria and tetanus.

Table 1.2: Differences between live attenuated and inactivated vaccines

Characteristics	Live attenuated	Inactivated
1. Content	Attenuated living microorganisms	Inactivated micro-organisms/their part
2. Administration to individuals with compromised immunity	Contraindicated	Not contraindicated
3. Storage conditions	Stringent	Not stringent
4. Manufacturing	Difficult	Easy
5. Prolonged immunity usually with a single dose	Yes	Multiple doses required
6. Immunity produced	Prolonged	Short lived
7. Cost of production	More	Less
8. Type of immunity produced	Cell mediated	Humoral

4. COMBINATIONS

Several serotypes of the same disease causing micro-organism **(polyvalent vaccines)** or antigens of various different diseases are combined together **(combined vaccines)** to provide for simultaneous administration and protection against various diseases. The combination can include various types of vaccines together such as in DPT Hib Polio Hep B combination vaccine, the vaccines included are toxoids (DT), subunit protein (pertussis), protein conjugate (Hib), recombinant DNA vaccine (Hep B) and inactivated vaccine (polio). Similarly, polio vaccine contains three serotypes and pneumococcal vaccine provides protection against 23 serotypes of the same disease causing microorganism.

Immunoglobulins

- Immunoglobulins provide "passive" or ready-made immunity to the individual. They can be prepared from non-human sources such as animals, usually horses or from human sources.
- When prepared from non-human sources, they are known as antiserum. Administration of antisera can lead to acute reactions such as serum sickness or anaphylaxis. They should therefore be tested intradermally before administration.

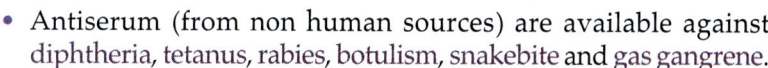

- Antiserum (from non human sources) are available against diphtheria, tetanus, rabies, botulism, snakebite and gas gangrene.
- Immunoglobulins obtained from human sources have lesser chances of reactions.
- Immunoglobulins/antiserum are costly; however they provide immediate protection and therefore are the mainstay of management against several infections following exposure.
- They should be administered as soon as possible following exposure.

They are very effective in
- Controlling outbreaks (hepatitis A)
- Providing immediate protection to immunosuppressed or susceptible contacts of diseased persons (varicella, hepatitis B, measles)
- Preventing the development of the disease in an exposed person (hepatitis B, hepatitis C, rubella, rabies, tetanus and Rh incompatibility).

Some Important Points to be Remembered about Vaccination

- There are several preventive and control measures which are to be followed for the prevention and control of vaccine preventable diseases. Immunization is one of them. Immunization is used as a preventive measure "along with" other control measures. Immunization alone is usually ineffective in preventing or controlling the disease. Moreover, since the vaccination is not 100% effective, administration of vaccine cannot guarantee prevention from the disease.
- Interruption of the recommended schedules with a delay between doses does not interfere with the final immunity achieved nor does it necessitate starting the series of vaccination all over again, regardless of the length of time elapsed between doses. So, a child who is supposed to receive DPT vaccine at 6, 10 and 14 weeks does not turn up at 10 weeks for receiving the second dose but instead arrives at the age of 6 months, should be given the 2nd dose at 6 months and called one month later for the 3rd dose. There is no need to restart the vaccination schedule. However, it is important to remember that the minimum interval between two vaccines or two doses of the vaccine should be at least 4 weeks. An exception to this rule is

the interval between the pulse polio doses of OPV and the routine vaccines. A child should be given the pulse polio vaccine doses irrespective of the fact that he/she has received the routine vaccines within the last one month or is due for the vaccines in the next one month.

- When multiple vaccines are to be given simultaneously
    - Give them maximum within 24 hours, preferably simultaneously
    - Administer at different sites or at least 1 inch apart. If a vaccine and immunoglobulin are administered simultaneously, give them at different anatomic sites to prevent interference.
    - Do not mix different vaccines in the same syringe or vial unless indicated by the manufacturer; instead use a combination vaccine if available.
- Age of vaccination when indicated means "completed age".
- Minimum interval between two vaccines is 4 weeks (–4 days can be allowed).
- Beneficiaries should be observed for 15–20 minutes following immunization for any allergic reaction. Some individuals experience fainting attacks following administration of injection. So as a precaution all individuals specially adolescents and adults should be made to lie down after injection for 10–15 minutes to prevent the falls and injuries resulting due to these fainting attacks.
- In immunocompromised individuals, all inactivated vaccines can be given. However, live vaccines should not be given to those with severe immunodeficiency. Household contacts of patients with immunodeficiency should not be given vaccines that can be transmitted from one to another, such as OPV. However, other live vaccines, which are not transmissible, can be given safely and definitely to the household contacts. The site of injection should not be cleaned by a spirit swab before administration of a live attenuated vaccine since live attenuated vaccine components may get destroyed if they come in contact with the spirit. If the injection site requires cleaning with the spirit, it should be allowed to dry up before injecting the vaccine.
- The swab should be moved in circular direction from inside out while cleaning the injection site.

- Different swabs should be used for cleaning the site before vaccination and stopping the oozing of blood after vaccination.
- If an unvaccinated child comes to the immunization clinic for the first time at a later age than what is recommended/scheduled, he/she may be given all the vaccines simultaneously at different sites. For example if a child comes at the age of 4 months for the first time, he/she may be given BCG, first dose of DPT, hepatitis B and OPV simultaneously and called after 4 weeks for the next dose.
- If the parent is not willing for simultaneous administration of all the vaccines, the vaccine which is due for that particular age may be given first and the rest may be given at a later date. For e.g. if a child comes at 9 months of age and the parents are not willing for administration of all the vaccines (BCG, DPT, OPV, Hep B and measles), measles should be given as a priority and the rest of the vaccines may be given after 4 weeks.

The description of immunizing agents in this book is being discussed under following common headings:

- *Type of vaccine:* Such as live, killed, subunit.
- *Indications* for administration of vaccine
- *Age* of administration
- *Dose:* It is usually 0.5 ml for IM/SC injections.
- *Site:* Gluteal region should NOT be used for IM injections to prevent injury to sciatic nerve. It also inhibits absorption due to increased fatty tissue.

Note: Site refers to the part of the body on which the vaccine is administered, i.e. deltoid, gluteal; whereas route refers to the mode/method of administration, i.e. intramuscular, intradermal, subcutaneous or oral.

- *Route*
  - Intradermal: BCG and rabies
  - Subcutaneous (S/c) route for measles, MMR, varicella, meningococcal polysaccharide, JE, yellow fever.
  - SC/IM: Pneumococcal polysaccharide and IPV
  - Intramuscular (IM): Rest of the vaccines
- *Number of doses and schedule:* Schedule refers to the period of gap between the number of doses such as 0, 1, 6 for hepatitis B.
- *Contraindications:* Includes absolute and relative contraindications.

- *Adverse effects:* A medical incident that takes place after vaccination causes concern and is believed to be caused by immunization. It is important to inform the parents about the impending adverse effects that are a sequelae to vaccination (such as fever after DPT) to avoid any panic. It is discussed in more detail later. Vaccine efficacy calculated as:

$$\frac{\text{Attack rate in unvaccinated population} - \text{Attack rate in vaccinated population}}{\text{Attack rate in unvaccinated population}} \times 100$$

- *Vaccine effectiveness:* Depends on vaccine efficacy and herd effect which is defined as reduction of infection in the unimmunized population as a result of immunizing a proportion of population. Tetanus and BCG vaccines have no herd effect. Conjugated pneumococcal and Hib vaccines have good herd effect.
- Vaccine efficacy and effectiveness are obtained from field studies in different population groups.

SOME FREQUENTLY ASKED QUESTIONS (FAQs)

Q. What is your opinion about the vaccines and other pharmaceutical agents? Is there any difference between them?

Ans. A vaccine is "a biological preparation" that improves immunity to a particular disease. A vaccine typically contains an agent that resembles a disease-causing microorganism, and is often made from weakened or killed forms of the microbe, its toxins or one of its surface proteins. In contrast, a drug is a chemical substance. When compared to drugs, vaccines are delicate substances that lose potency if they are exposed to temperatures that are too warm or too cold. It is useless to vaccinate a child if the vaccine that was used is exposed to high or low temperature than recommended

Q. What do you mean by word "attenuation"?

Ans. The word 'attenuation' literally means 'weak'. When it is used for a vaccine, it means that the vaccine virus is so weak that it is unable to cause the disease but is able to act as an antigen, which leads to the production of the antibodies by the body's immune system.

Q. How is the live attenuated vaccine produced?

Ans. In a live attenuated vaccine, the virus is attenuated by passage through the cells of foreign host which could be embryonated eggs or cells of live animals or through tissue culture, etc. After introduction into these cells, virus mutates. This mutation leads to growth of viruses in the foreign cells and the strain of the virus produced is completely different from the original one. This strain is able to produce the antibodies in the host cells but is unable to cause the disease (attenuated virus) and therefore this attenuated virus is used in the production of vaccine.

Q. How are the killed/inactivated vaccines produced?

Ans. The killed vaccines are inactivated vaccines where the microorganisms, like bacteria or viruses are killed by physical/chemical process but the capsid or the part of bacteria is well recognized by the immune system. Therefore, when they are introduced in the body they are unable to reproduce, but able to act as antigen for production of antibodies.

Q. Boosters are required frequently for which types of vaccines and why?

Ans. Boosters are frequently required for killed/inactivated vaccines/toxoids since the microorganism is not able to reproduce thereby necessitating frequent boosters to maintain the immunity. Some live attenuated vaccines administered through oral route such as OPV and Rotavirus also require boosters because they are lost through the digestive tract.

Q. What are the other components of a vaccine apart from the antigen?

Ans. Vaccines have various other components apart from the antigen such as:
1. Adjuvants
2. Preservatives
3. Antibiotics
4. Stabilizers

Adjuvants are substances added to **enhance the immuno-genicity** of the vaccine. These include salts of aluminum such as aluminum hydroxide in hepatitis A and B vaccine, human papillomavirus vaccine, DPT, etc. Other adjuvants used are tween 80, aluminum phosphate, squalene, alpha tocopherol, etc.

Preservatives are added to vaccines to **prevent the contamination** of killed or subunit vaccines by viruses, bacteria etc. It is therefore prevents infections due to the contaminated vaccines. Vaccines which do not have preservatives (BCG, measles, etc.) should be used within the stipulated time period or else should be discarded.

Antibiotics also prevent bacterial contamination, but as against the preservatives, this protection is afforded during the process of manufacturing, rather than after production.

Stabilizers, as the name suggests, are added to stabilize the vaccine so that they do not lose their potency due to alteration in pH, freeze drying, etc. Commonly used stabilizers include human and bovine serum albumin, potassium or sodium salts, lactose, etc.

Q. Should a child be immunized if the child's mother is pregnant?

Ans. Yes, pregnancy does not pose a contraindication to routine vaccine administration to a child.

Q. Should a child having chronic disease be immunized?

Ans. Usually, children with chronic diseases do not pose a contraindication (except if child is having decreased immunity) to routine vaccine administration. In fact, they should be given priority in offering the vaccine.

Q. Can we vaccinate to a child who is allergic?

Ans. Yes, diseases like asthma or allergies are not contraindications to any vaccine. However, since some of the vaccines are prepared using egg therefore an important contraindication for some of the vaccines is severe egg allergy.

Q. What do you think is better-natural immunity or vaccine induced immunity?

Ans. The vaccine-induced immunity may diminish with time but the 'natural' immunity, acquired by catching the disease, is usually lifelong. However, this does not mean that we should wait for natural infection to occur, as the disadvantage with natural infection or disease is that it can kill or leave a child permanently handicapped and contribute to sickness absenteeism in schools. On the other hand, vaccines are many times safer than the diseases they prevent and moreover children or adults can be re-immunized if their immunity from the vaccines falls to a low level.

Q. Can administering too many vaccines overload the immune system?

Ans. No, there is no evidence that too many vaccines overload the immune system.

Q. In recent years, diseases like polio, tetanus, whooping cough and diphtheria have already declined significantly or disappeared from most parts of India. So, shall we stop offering these vaccines to our children against these diseases?

Ans. Though, these diseases are much less common now, but the bacteria and viruses that cause them are still present. The fact is reinforced by the appearance of diseases where vaccination rates have declined. Therefore, it is advisable to vaccinate the children according to the National Immunization Programme.

Q. Do breastfed children need a different vaccination schedule?

Ans. No. breastfed children should be vaccinated according to the standard schedule. Breast milk, especially colostrum contains small amounts of antibodies, but these do not interfere with the immunization process.

Q. What vaccines do you give to a child with no immunization records?

Ans. If there is no satisfactory verbal or written record of immunization, the child should be given immunizations from then on as if they were never immunized previously.

Q. What are false contraindications to vaccine administration?

Ans. The incorrect reasons for withholding a vaccine are called "false contraindications". The list below comprises some examples

of false contraindications. If an infant or adult presents with any of these, they should be vaccinated.

- Minor illnesses such as upper respiratory infections, or diarrhea or fever < 38.5°C
- Allergy, asthma or other atopic manifestations such as hay fever or snuffles
- Prematurity/LBW
- Malnutrition
- Infant being breastfed
- Family history of convulsions
- Treatment with antibiotics, low dose corticosteroids or locally acting steroids
- Dermatoses, eczema or localized skin infection
- Chronic diseases of the heart, lung, kidney and liver
- Stable neurological conditions, such as cerebral palsy and Down syndrome
- History of jaundice after birth

Q. What are the recommendations of IAP for catch up of some common vaccines in adolescents?

Ans. Recommendations of IAP for catch-up immunization (if the vaccination schedule has not been started/completed) in adolescents is as follows:

MMR	2 doses at an interval of 4–8 weeks
Varicella	2 doses at an interval of 4–8 weeks
Hepatitis A	2 doses at 0 and 6 months
Hepatitis B	3 doses at 0, 1, 6 m
Typhoid	One dose repeated at a minimum interval of three years
Influenza	One dose every year
JE	One dose upto 15 years of age
Pneumococcal	Two doses at an interval of 5 years
HPV	3 doses in pre-adolescent age after 9 years

Q. Which vaccines are required to be administered in travelers?

Ans. Vaccines required for selective use in travelers are:
- Hepatitis A

- Typhoid fever
- Rabies
- Cholera
- Japanese encephalitis
- Tick-borne encephalitis
- Meningococcal disease
- Yellow fever

Q. What are combination vaccines?

Ans. *Combination vaccines*
- When antigens/serotypes of different diseases are combined together into a single vaccine, it is known as combination vaccine.
- When they contain different serotypes of the same pathogen, they are known as bivalent (containing two serotypes) or polyvalent/ multivalent (more than 2 serotypes)
- When they contain antigens of different pathogens they are known as combined/combination vaccines.
- Certain vaccine products have to be mixed or reconstituted before administration. Such vaccine products are labeled with a slash (/) between the names of the vaccines.
- Products with a dash (–) in between the vaccine products do not require to be mixed or reconstituted and can be used straightaway after drawing from the vial.

Advantages
- It reduces the number of injections and the number of contact/ visits to the health care system.
- It also reduces the cost of cold chain maintenance for the vaccines and record maintenance

Disadvantages
- It might increase the rates of adverse events
- It may also modify the immunogenicity of the vaccine components
- It may also reduce the shelf life of the vaccines as compared to the individual vaccines.

Combination vaccines available
- DPT (Diphtheria, pertussis, tetanus)
- DTwP (Diphtheria, Tetanus, whole cell pertussis)
- DTaP (diphtheria, tetanus, acellular pertussis)
- DTwP+ Hep B
- DTwP+ Hib, DTwP+ Hib + Hep B (these combinations are available as ready to use vaccines or in lyophilized forms, in which Hib is to be reconstituted with other vaccines in the pack from same manufacturer)
- DTaP+Hib (lyophilized forms), DTaP + Hib + IPV (ready to use formulations), DTaP/Hep B
- MMR (measles, mumps, rubella)
- MMRV vaccine (measles, mumps, rubella, varicella)
- Oral polio vaccine (polyvalent-3 serotypes/two serotypes depending on the need)
- Inactivated polio vaccine (polyvalent)
- Hepatitis A + hepatitis B

2

Safe Injection Practices

Since vaccination involves a medical intervention in the form of an injection, it includes a certain risk of transmission of blood-borne infections such as HIV, hepatitis B, hepatitis C, etc. Therefore practicing safe injection procedures will ensure safety from transmission of infection due to contaminated syringes to:

- Person who is administering the vaccine
- Person receiving it
- Person disposing it
- Scavengers
- General public.

Following are some of the important points to be considered for ensuring safety from injections during vaccination session:

I. Use Sterile Injection Equipment

- Please ensure that the syringe and needle is from a sealed and undamaged packaging (either during transport or storage or by moisture/heat, etc.).
- Check for the expiry date of the package of syringe and needle.

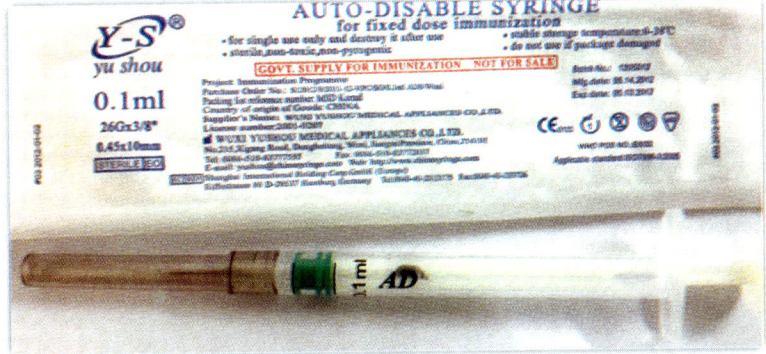

- The package should be opened in front of the patient and every injection should be given by using a new syringe and needle.
- AD syringes (autodisable syringes), which are now provided under the immunization programme should be used for vaccination. These are syringes that get locked after a single use and therefore cannot be reused again. This substantially reduces the chances of transmission of blood-borne infections from one person to another.

II. Prevent Contamination at the Vaccination Site

- Wash hands thoroughly using soap and running water or alcohol based preparation before and after vaccination session.
- In case of withdrawing vaccine from multi-dose vials, always pierce the septum with a sterile needle. Never leave a needle in the vial. Remove needles from multi-dose vials between injections. Use single dose vials rather than multi-dose vials, if possible to prevent contamination.
- Swabbing of clean vial tops or ampoules with an antiseptic or disinfectant is not necessary. If swabbing is required, use a clean, single-use swab rather than using the same swab again and again.
- Although glass ampoules have now been phased out from immunization programme, however, if it is to be opened, use a clean protective barrier (e.g. small gauze pad or cotton ball) when opening it. Do not open glass ampoules with bare fingers or break it with any other object as the glass pieces may get scattered and cause injury.
- The expiry date of the vaccines should be checked before administration. The vaccines should also be inspected for visible contamination, cracks, or leaks and the status of VVM.
- Observe if a needle touches any non-sterile surface (e.g. hands).
- If the vaccine vials, especially the septum are submerged in water, they should be discarded as there is a possibility of contamination.

III. Maintain the Effectiveness and Safety of Vaccines

- Confirm the vaccine to be given from the immunization card.
- Check for product-specific recommendations for use, storage and handling of vaccine preparations.

- Use diluent from the same manufacturer while reconstituting the vaccines. Nowadays, the vaccines, diluents, syringes and safety boxes are supplied together as a package to ensure that all the essential equipment and supplies for vaccination are in sufficient and appropriate amount. This is known as "bundling".
- Mark the time of reconstitution of vaccines and ensure that it is not used beyond the stipulated time period (3 hrs for BCG and 4 hrs for measles).

IV. Administering Injections

- If the integrity of the skin of the vaccinator is compromised by any infectious skin conditions, he/she should avoid giving injections. If there are small cuts on the hand, they should be covered and gloves should be worn.
- Gloves should be worn in case of open lesions on hands/ potential contact with body fluids by the vaccinator.
- Swabbing of clean skin by spirit is unnecessary as it may kill the microorganisms in the live attenuated vaccines.
- If the skin is to be swabbed with an antiseptic, a clean, separate single-use swab should be used before giving injection and after the injection for cleaning the blood that is oozing out from the injection site. Do not use the same swab both before and after the injection.
- Do not touch the hub or shaft of the needle (which is usually practiced by vaccinators for increasing the stability of the syringe) while drawing vaccine or administering it, especially during the administration of intradermal injection of BCG.
- Do not pre-fill the vaccine in the syringe so as to prevent administration errors.
- Communicate with the parents regarding the vaccine reactions that may happen after the injection.

V. Prevent Needle Stick Injuries to the Provider

- Anticipate and take measures to prevent sudden patient movement during and after injection.
- The instructions for part preparation of the child should be given before loading the vaccine in the syringe. The part preparation should not be done after loading the vaccine, since

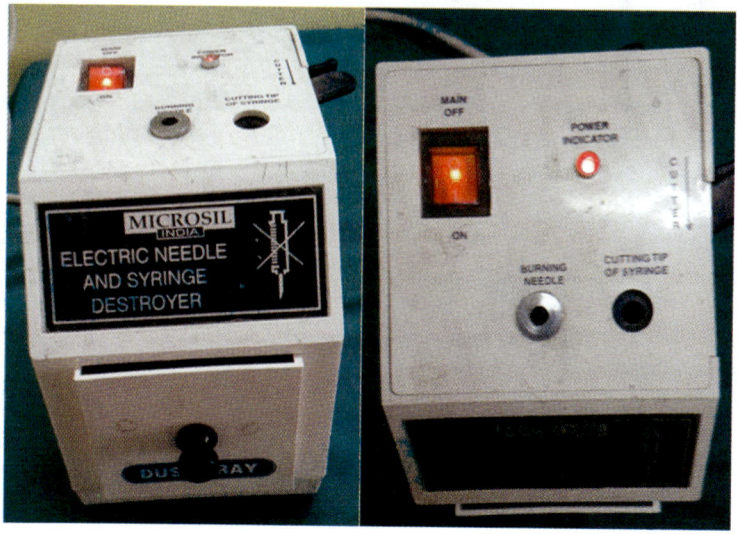

Needle and syringe destroyer from front and top

the child may hit the syringe when you attempt to prepare the child for vaccination.

- Do not recap disposable, single use needles and syringes after giving injections. Not with one hand, not with two, not at all!
- Discard the needle and syringe immediately by using the needle cutter/destroyer and puncture proof boxes;
- Do not use boxes that are open, overflowing or punctured. Get a new one!
- Seal safety boxes before they are completely full. Do not overfill the puncture proof box and never try to press the syringes in the box to accommodate more syringes as this will increase the chances of injury.
- The syringes should be destroyed in the needle destroyer and disposed by the vaccinator himself/herself and should not be given to any other person for destruction and disposal
- Cut the needle from the hub; not shaft. Remember, the equipment for destroying the syringe is known as hub cutter; not shaft cutter.
- Do not collect the syringes on the table for collective disposal. This is a very common practice during the immunization sessions, because of the high number of beneficiaries which does not provide enough time to the vaccinator for proper disposal of the syringes.

3

Adverse Events Following Immunization (AEFI)

It is a medical incident that takes place after vaccination, causes concern and is believed to be caused by immunization. Monitoring of AEFI and action taken in response to it is very important in the National Immunization Programme, to maintain the faith of the people in the vaccination programme.

AEFI are classified under following headings:

1. *Vaccine product related reaction*
- Event caused by the vaccine, e.g. vaccine associated paralytic polio (VAPP) following administration of OPV; or
- Precipitated by the vaccine even when given correctly, e.g. febrile seizure following vaccination in a predisposed child.
- It is caused by inherent properties of the vaccine.
- Proper communication regarding the possibility of vaccine reaction and counseling may be helpful in reducing the panic associated with the vaccine reactions. Appropriate medications may be prescribed beforehand during vaccination, such as paracetamol for fever after DPT vaccination, for controlling the vaccine reaction.

2. *Vaccine quality defect related reaction:* Event caused by defect in the vaccine product or the administration device

3. *Immunization error related reaction/programme error:* Event caused by an error in vaccine storage, transport, preparation, handling, or administration, e.g. deaths following measles vaccination due to toxic shock syndrome resulting from improper reconstitution and storage of measles vaccine is the most recent example. Programme errors lead to loss of faith of people in the immunization programme which leads to huge loss of health of the people.

4. *Immunization anxiety related reaction/injection reaction:* Event from anxiety about, or pain from, the *injection itself rather than the vaccine.* Examples include syncope due to pain of

vaccination, injection site abscesses, sciatic nerve damage due to gluteal injection. Choosing the right site and using the right method of giving injection may reduce injection reactions due to faulty techniques or wrong site.

5. *Coincidental:* Event that happens after immunization but *not caused by the vaccine*—a chance association. Example is the association between immunization and sudden infant death syndrome (SIDS or cot death), as the incidence of SIDS peaks around the age when infant immunizations are delivered.

6. *Unknown:* The cause of the event cannot be determined.

- Of all these types of AEFI, programme error is preventable to quite an extent; the rest of the AEFI can be tackled by appropriate counseling and interventions to reduce the effect. All the maintenance of cold chain and monitoring and supervision of vaccination sessions are basically aimed at reducing the programme errors.
- The specific vaccine reactions are listed along with the description of individual vaccines in the specific chapters.

FAQs

Q. Can we do a sensitivity testing for adverse reaction in a child before giving him a vaccine?

Ans. Sensitivity testing is not usually done for vaccines and if done would not yield reliable results as the site of vaccination may vary in sensitivity testing (intradermal) and actual vaccine administration (Intradermal/subcutaneous/intramuscular/oral).

Q. Is there any genetic predisposition to adverse effects? Can the sibling of a child who has had an adverse effect to a vaccine, be vaccinated safely?

Ans. Genetic predisposition to adverse effect has not been documented and the siblings can be vaccinated safely.

Q. If there is a serious adverse reaction to a previous dose of vaccine, can the next dose be administered under the cover of medications?

Ans. The subsequent doses of the vaccine which had lead to a serious adverse effect should *never* be given, not even under the cover of medications.

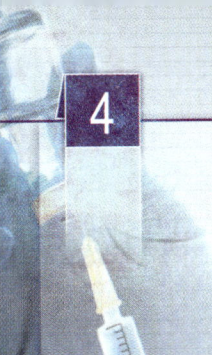

4

Cold Chain

Q. What is cold chain?

Ans. Immunization is one of the most effective ways of preventing diseases in a population. Though it seems very simple to give a vaccine to a child but if we explore the actual process of vaccination retrospectively then we will be able to appreciate the complexity of the whole system by which a child is vaccinated. This whole system includes a crucial component known as "Cold chain".

The cold chain is a "system of transporting, storing and distributing the vaccine at recommended temperature from the site of manufacturer to the actual vaccination site".

The vaccine travels through the following points in the cold chain system to reach the beneficiaries:

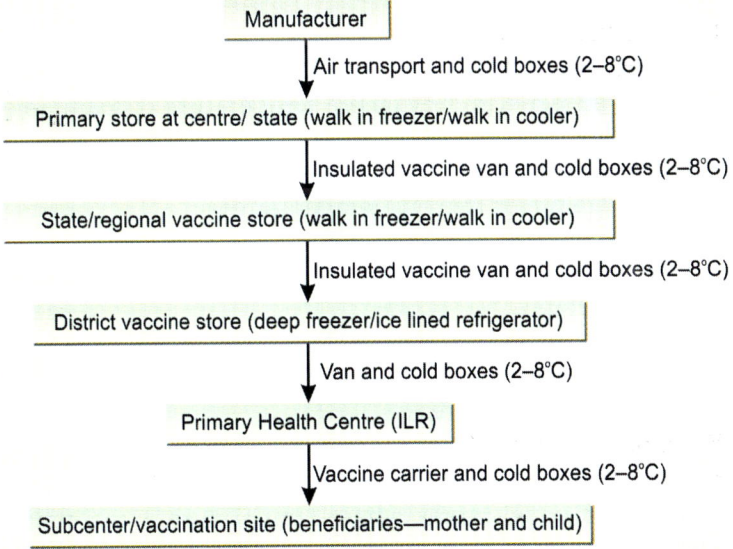

```
                    Manufacturer
                         │ Air transport and cold boxes (2–8°C)
                         ▼
   Primary store at centre/ state (walk in freezer/walk in cooler)
                         │ Insulated vaccine van and cold boxes (2–8°C)
                         ▼
   State/regional vaccine store (walk in freezer/walk in cooler)
                         │ Insulated vaccine van and cold boxes (2–8°C)
                         ▼
   District vaccine store (deep freezer/ice lined refrigerator)
                         │ Van and cold boxes (2–8°C)
                         ▼
              Primary Health Centre (ILR)
                         │ Vaccine carrier and cold boxes (2–8°C)
                         ▼
   Subcenter/vaccination site (beneficiaries—mother and child)
```

Q. Why it is called a "Cold chain"?

Ans. Since it is a system or chain of various equipment by which vaccine is kept at a "lower/cold temperature" (usually 2–8°C) right from the production to the actual vaccination site, it is known as 'Cold chain'. This temperature maintenance is essential because the vaccines are heat/freeze sensitive and may lose their potency on exposure to higher or lower temperatures.

Q. What are the elements of a cold chain?

Ans. *Cold chain elements:* There are following elements in the cold chain:

1. *Personnel:* People involved in managing the vaccine distribution.
2. *Equipment* involved in storage and transport of vaccine.
3. *Transport facilities:* Refrigerated vehicles
4. *Maintenance of equipment.*
5. *Monitoring* of the system from time to time.

Q. What are the cold chain equipment?

Ans. *Cold chain equipment*

We can serially divide the cold chain equipment into following components from higher to lower center.

a. *Walk in freezer (WIF)*
   - These are prefabricated modular polyurethane (PUF) insulated panel rooms where temperature is maintained from 0 to –20°C.
   - These are called as WIF since you can 'walk' inside the room which maintains freezing temperatures.
   - These rooms are installed with refrigeration units and with temperature meter and alarm system for proper maintenance of temperature.
   - These are used for storing OPV and frozen ice packs at state or regional level and the usual storing capacity is from 15 to 20 lakh doses or more.

b. *Walk in cold rooms (WIC rooms)*
   - These are prefabricated modular polyurethane (PUF) insulated panel rooms where temperature is maintained from +2 to +8°C.

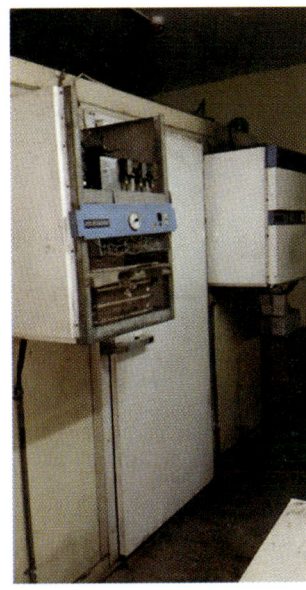

**Refrigeration units and door
of walk-in-cold (WIC) room**

- They are also located at state or regional level and can serve 4–5 districts.
- These are used for storing DPT, DT, TT, BCG, measles, Hep B vaccines, etc. at state or regional level and the usual storing capacity is from 12 to 15 lakh doses or more.

c. *Deep freezers (300/ 286/ 140/ 116 liter capacity)*

- These are top opening lid refrigerators and are available at district level.
- These are used for making ice packs and to store OPV vaccines.
- A large deep freezer (DF) can store 200 ice packs or 1,20,000 –1,80,000 doses of OPV (the stock for about 3 months).
- The small deep freezer can store 100 ice packs.
- The temperature is maintained from –15 to –25°C.
- The hold over time for deep freezer is 18 hours and 22 hrs at 43°C and 32°C respectively.
- At PHC level, DF is not used for storing vaccines; they are used for making ice packs only.

d. *Ice lined refrigerator (ILR) (300/ 200/ 140 and 70 liters)*

- These are also top opening lid refrigerators whose work is to maintain temperature between +2 and + 8°C and are used to store vaccines usually at CHC and PHC levels.

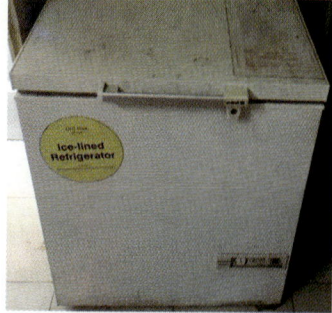
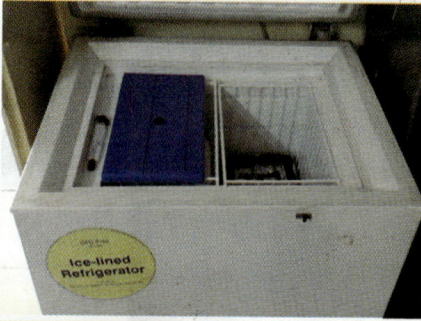
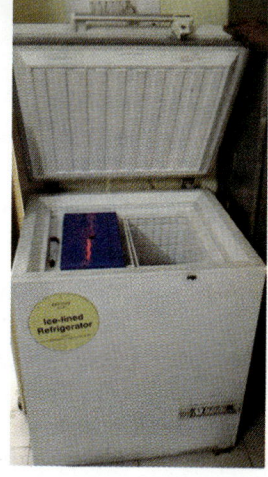

- The vaccines should not be stored beyond 1 month at PHC.
- The vaccine storage capacity: 300 liters of ILR has the capacity to store 60,000 doses of vaccine and 140 liters can store 25,000 doses.
- All the vaccines must be kept in the basket in ILR and none of the vaccines should be placed directly on the floor of ILR so as to prevent the freezing of vaccines.
- Proper spacing should be provided in between the boxes for air circulation.
- A dial thermometer/stem thermometer should be kept in the ILR and temperature should be recorded twice a day.

e. *Cold boxes (20 or 5 liters)*
   - Cold boxes are insulated containers lined with ice packs on the inside walls and floor to maintain a temperature between +2°C and +8°C.

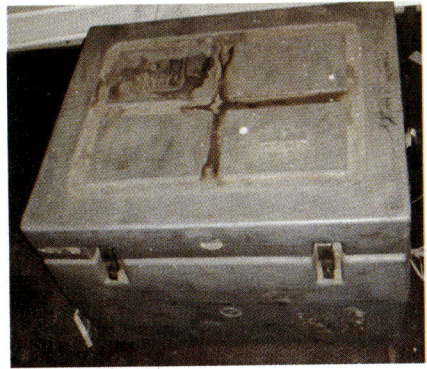
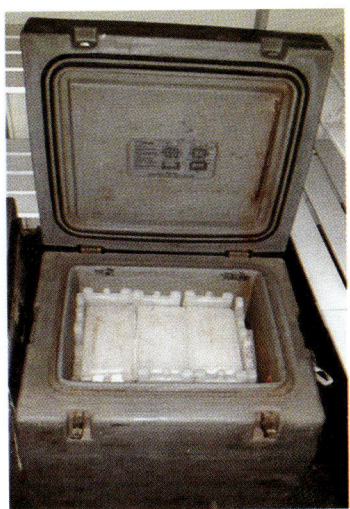

Outer and inner view of a small cold box

- They are used to collect and transport vaccine supplies from State to Regional Vaccine Stores and/or District Vaccine Stores and/or to PHC.
- Hold over time of cold boxes is 6.5 days and 10 days at 43°C and 32°C respectively, which is the maximum among all equipment.
- Cold boxes are supplied to all peripheral centers for transport of vaccines.
- The vials should not be placed in direct contact with the frozen ice packs.
- The large box can store 6000 doses of vaccines with 50 ice packs, whereas the small box can store 1500 doses with 24 ice packs.

f. *Vaccine carriers (1.7 liters):* Vaccine carriers are insulated boxes used to carry small quantities of vaccines (16–20 vials). They are lined with four ice packs on the inside to maintain the temperature between +2°C and +8°C. The hold over time of vaccine carrier is 34 hours and 51 hours at 43°C and 32°C respectively.

g. *Ice packs:* These are plastic containers filled with water and frozen for use. They are used to line the cold boxes and vaccine carriers during transport of vaccines and help in maintaining the temperature to optimum level (+2°C to +8°C). The ice packs

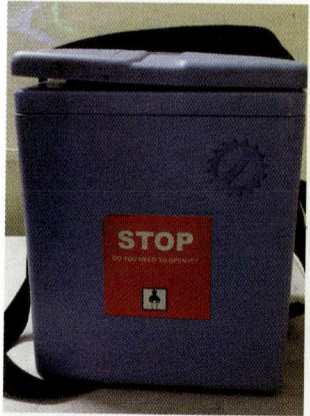

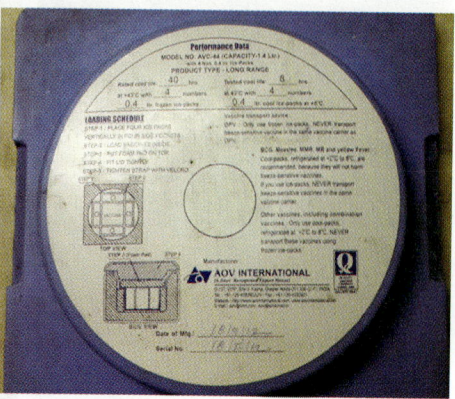

Outer view of vaccine carrier   Inner view of lid of vaccine carrier

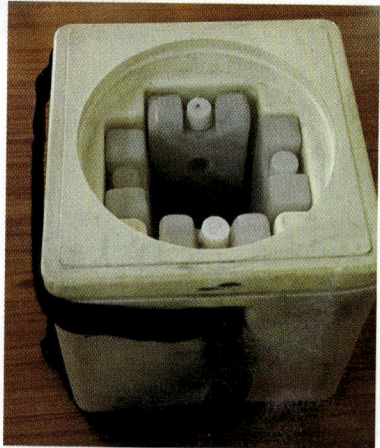

Inner view of vaccine carrier

are placed vertically in the DF, sides of cold boxes and vaccine carriers. The T series vaccines should not be kept in direct contact with the ice packs; they should be wrapped in a cardboard or placed in a plastic packet/box and then placed inside the cold box or vaccine carrier.

h. *Vaccine vans:* They are insulated vans provided at district level for transportation of vaccines from the regional or state stores. They can transport approximately 6–10 lakh doses

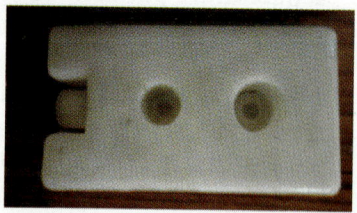

of mixed antigens at a time. The vaccines are transported in cold boxes in the vaccine vans.

Remember

- The optimum temperature of all the cold chain equipment is between +2°C and +8°C, except deep freezer and WIF which maintain a temperature between –15°C and –25°C.
- The maximum hold over time is that of cold box, which is quite logical, because the vaccines have to be kept in the cold boxes for a longer period of time during transport.

Q. What is the difference between ILR and normal/home refrigerators?

Ans. ILR has an ice bank (ice packed lining) which keeps the internal temperature at a safe level despite electricity failure. Hold over time (time required for a well functioning cold chain equipment to reach the safe higher limit of temperature from the lower limit, i.e. from 2°C to 8°C, in the absence of electrical supply) of ILR is up to 62 hours and 78 hours at 43°C and 32°C respectively; while home refrigerators are able to maintain the temperature for only 4 hours during electricity failure. Moreover since the ILR is top opening therefore the speed of exit of cold air from the ILR is less as compared to home refrigerators.

Q. Why ice packs should not be 100% filled with water?

Ans. Ice packs are not fully filled with water so as to allow for expansion as water freezes. If they are filled 100%, they might crack on freezing due to expansion. They are filled till the "neck".

Q. How will you asses that ice pack is fully frozen?

Ans. The assessment of ice pack to ensure that it is fully frozen is made by rock solid feel and stony sound which is produced if we leave it from some height on the ground. However, before putting it in the vaccine carrier, ice packs are 'conditioned' (also known as "thawing effect") i.e. kept at room temperature to allow drops to appear on the ice packs, to prevent the freezing of the vaccines during transport by exposure to subzero temperature.

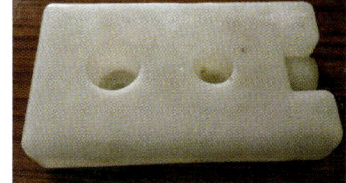

Q. Which thermometers should be preferably used in ILR and deep refrigerators for monitoring the temperature?

Ans. Generally we use dial/stem thermometers for monitoring the temperature of the cold chain equipment. Ideally, alcohol thermometers should be used to measure the temperature in both ILR and deep freezer, as they are more sensitive and accurate and they can record temperatures from –50°C to +50°C. Dial thermometers need to be calibrated at periodic intervals. The reading of the thermometer should be taken while it is placed inside the cold chain equipment; not by taking it out. Temperature is recorded twice a day and record is maintained in a log book.

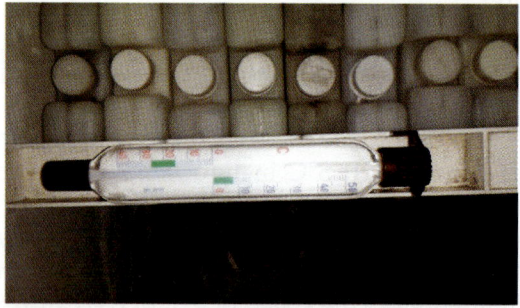

Stem thermometer placed inside the deep freezer

Q. At which place are there greater chances of cold chain failure?

Ans. The risk of cold chain failure is greatest at sub-center and village level due to the interrupted power supply and lack of knowledge and training regarding maintenance of temperature. For this reason, vaccines are not stored at the sub-center level and must be supplied on the day of vaccination.

Q. Which vaccine can be stored at subcentre level?

Ans. No vaccine should be stored at sub-center level. It is supplied to the sub-center on the day of vaccination.

Q. Where should the diluents, supplied along with the vaccine, be stored?

Ans. The diluents should ideally be stored along with the vaccine with which it is supplied. However due to shortage of space in cold chain equipment, diluents may be stored at room temperature, but it should be brought to the same temperature as that of the vaccine by keeping it with the vaccine for 24 hours before reconstitution, to prevent sudden rise of temperature of the vaccine during and after the reconstitution, thereby leading to a breakdown in the "cold chain".

Q. What should be done to the vaccine vials not opened during vaccination session?

Ans. The vaccines not opened during vaccination session should be taken back to the PHC and stored at the recommended temperature. They should be marked as "Returned unused" so that they are used "first" in the next session. The VVM of the vaccine should be checked for ensuring the maintenance of temperature. Vaccines that have been returned unused thrice should be discarded.

Q. What are the do's and don'ts to be followed for WIF/WIC?

Ans. Following is the list of do's and don'ts to be followed for proper maintenance of WIF/WIC:

Do's	Don'ts
• Keep the vaccines on the shelves only and allow space for the circulation of air between the boxes of vials	• The power supply to the rooms should be maintained continuously through the provision of an automatic generator system
• Follow the policy of early expiry first out (EEFO)	• The rooms should never be over loaded
• Only OPV should be stored in WIF; the rest of the vaccines to be stored in WIC	• The vaccines should not be stored on the floor
• Temperature should be recorded twice daily and record should be maintained	
• Maintain a log book	
• Restrict the entry to the WIF/WIC by allowing only authorized personnel, who should wear warm clothes while entering the rooms	

Q. What are the do's and don'ts to be followed for proper maintenance of the deep freezers and ILR?

Ans. Following is the list of do's and don'ts to be followed for proper maintenance of the deep freezers and ILR:

Do's	Don'ts
• They should be placed in a cool, dry, flat area on wooden platform and should be protected from direct sunlight or water	• Do not place heavy objects on the DF/ILR
• The equipment should be kept at a distance of at least 10 cm from the walls	• Do not sit on the DF/ILR
• They should be connected to the power socket permanently and should be labeled "Do not switch off or unplug"	• Do not use them for storing any other objects such as water bottles, medicines, eatables, etc.
• The equipment should be connected to a voltage stabilizer	• Do not open the equipment unnecessarily
• Temperature should be recorded twice a day and record maintained. Read the thermometer, where it is placed, not by taking it out	• Do not keep unusable vaccines (expired, frozen, VVM in unusable stage, etc.) in the DF/ILR
• The vaccines and the ice packs should be stacked properly to allow for air circulation and prevent freezing of freeze sensitive vaccines	• Do not store diluents in DF
• The equipment should be locked and keys should be available with designated personnel only	• Do not keep more than one months' supply at PHC and more than 3 months supply at district level.
• Defrost periodically when the frost on the walls is more than 5 mm, and clean the equipment after shifting the vaccines in the cold boxes.	• In case of breakdown, immediately shift the vaccines in the cold boxes and initiate remedial measures
• Mention the contact number of persons who are to be contacted in case of breakdown/ emergency	

Q. What are the do's and don'ts to be followed for proper maintenance of the cold boxes and vaccine carriers?

Ans. Following is the list of do's and don'ts to be followed for proper maintenance of the cold boxes and vaccine carriers:

Do's	Don'ts
• They must be dried after use as they may turn moldy if kept wet	• Never drop them on the ground as they may break and become leaky
• Store them in cool place as heat/ sunlight may cause cracks	• Never sit on them or place heavy objects on top of it.
• Always keep a thermometer in the cold box for monitoring of temperature	• Check periodically for any cracks and whether the rubber seal is in good condition.

Q. What is vaccine vial monitor (VVM)? (You frequently get to write a short note on VVM in your theory exams).

Ans. Vaccine vial monitor is used for monitoring heat sensitive vaccines. It is commonly present on the label of the vaccine vial and indicates the cumulative effect of rise of temperature of the vaccine above the critical point. Some vaccine vials have VVM on the cap to prevent it from getting wet and peeled off due to moisture. VVM undergoes changes through four sequential stages on exposure to heat as indicated below:

Stage 1: Inner square is white and outer circle is dark

Stage 2: Inner square is lighter than outer circle.

Stage 3: Inner square and outer circle are of the same color.

Stage 4: Inner square is darker than outer circle.

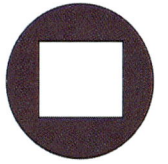 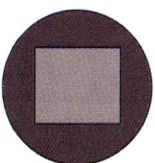 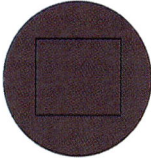 

Stage 1: Inner square is white and outer circle is dark.   **Stage 2**: Inner square is lighter than outer circle.   **Stage 3**: Inner square and outer circle are of the same color.   **Stage 4**: Inner square is darker than outer circle.

Usable stage: Can use the vaccine.   Un-usable stage: Cannot use the vaccine.

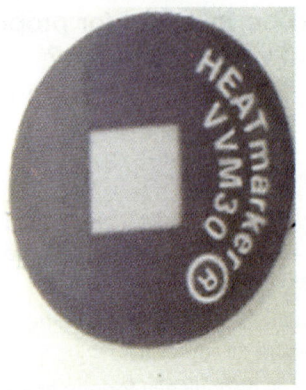

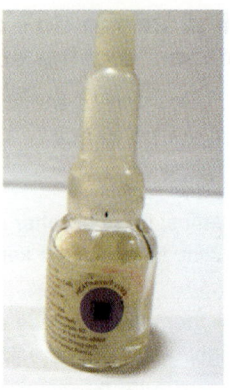

Stage 1 of VVM: Inner square is
white, outer circle is dark

Unusable stage of OPV: Inner square
is darker than the outer circle

Q. List down the heat sensitive vaccines in decreasing order.

Ans. Heat sensitivity of vaccines in **decreasing order**:

- BCG (after reconstitution)   (Most heat sensitive)
- Yellow fever   ↓
- OPV
- Measles
- DPT
- BCG (Before Reconstitution)
- DT, TT, Hepatitis B, JE   (Least heat sensitive)

Q. Which vaccines are sensitive to freezing?

Ans. Vaccines sensitive to freezing are as follows:

- T series vaccines (all vaccines with "T" in it.)
- Hepatitis B, DPT, DT, **TT**, HiB (Type B), diluent, hepatitis A, combination vaccines, HPV, IPV, inactivated influenza vaccines, meningococcal, Rotavirus, Typhoid, varicella vaccine.

Shake test: Used to test whether a freeze sensitive vaccine has been frozen at any point during transport/storage from manufacturer to the site of vaccination.

Procedure

1. Take a vaccine vial from the same lot/batch and same manufacturer, as that of "test" vaccine vial.

2. Ensure that this vial had not been frozen earlier. Label it as "control" to make sure that it is not used for vaccination in future. Freeze it and then thaw it.
3. Now take the "test" vaccine vial that is suspected to be frozen.
4. Hold both the vaccine vials between the index finger and thumb of a hand and shake it.
5. Then place both the vials upside down on a flat surface (since the sedimentation is visible better at the neck of the vial which does not have a label pasted on it) and observe the rate of sedimentation of the floccules.
6. If the rate of sedimentation in test vial is similar to or more than that in "control" vial, it indicates that the test vial had been frozen at some point of time during transport and storage.
7. It should then be discarded.

Freeze sensitive vaccines may also be monitored using freeze indicators such as **freeze watch** and **freeze tag**.

The vial in the **freeze watch** indicator releases the colored liquid when it is exposed to subzero temperatures for more than one hour.

Freeze tag has an alarm system which is visible as tick mark ("✓") if the vaccine has not been exposed to subzero temperature. The sign converts to a cross ("X") if the vaccine has been exposed to subzero temperature for more than one hour.

Q. What are the light sensitive vaccines?

Ans. The light sensitive vaccines are: Measles, BCG, MMR, measles-rubella and rubella. These vaccines are supplied in dark amber colored vials and need to be protected from sunlight as they may lose their potency.

5

National Immunization Schedule

The vaccines to be administered to children under National Immunization Schedule as per the age are given in Table 5.1:

Table 5.1: List of vaccines administered under National Immunization Schedule

Age	Vaccines	Diseases prevented	Route and site	Dose
At birth	BCG (can be given till 1 year)	Tuberculosis	Intradermal Left arm at insertion of deltoid	0.1 ml
	OPV (zero dose for institutional deliveries)	Poliomyelitis	Oral	2 drops
	Hep B (within 24 hrs)	Hepatitis B	IM, A/L aspect of mid thigh	0.5 ml
6, 10, 14 weeks	DPT	Diphtheria, pertussis, tetanus	IM, A/L aspect of mid thigh	0.5 ml
	OPV	Same as above		
	Hepatitis B or	Same as above		
	Pentavalent vaccines in selected states (DPT, Hep B and Hib)	Diphtheria, pertussis, tetanus, Hep B and Hib	IM, A/L aspect of mid thigh	0.5 ml
9–12 m	Measles	Measles	Subcutaneous, right arm	0.5 ml

Contd.

Table 5.1: List of vaccines administered under National Immunization Schedule (*Contd.*)

Age	Vaccines	Diseases prevented	Route and site	Dose
	Vitamin A 1st dose	Night blindness	Oral	1 ml (1 lakh unit)
	JE in selected districts	JE	Subcutaneous, right arm	0.5 ml
16–24 m	Measles 2nd dose	Same as above		
	DPT booster	Same as above		
	OPV booster	Same as above		
	JE in selected districts (6 m after vaccination drive)	Same as above		
	Vitamin A 2nd dose and subsequently every 6 months	Same as above		2 ml (2 lakh units)
5–6 yrs	DPT booster	Same as above		
10 and 16 yrs	Tetanus toxoid			
Pregnant woman	Tetanus toxoid 2 doses (only one dose if vaccinated in last 3 yrs)	Tetanus	IM, deltoid	0.5 ml

Note
- Age of administration refers to completed age.
- 6, 10 , 14 weeks can be better remembered and also advised to parents as 1.5, 2.5 and 3.5 months which is easier to remember by the parents.

New vaccines to be introduced in NIS as per National Technical Advisory Group on Immunization (NTAGI) recommendation:
- Injectable polio vaccine (IPV): As an additional dose along with 3rd dose of DPT (at 14th week) in the entire country in the first quarter of 2016.

- *Rotavirus vaccine:* Introduction of Rotavirus vaccine in Universal Immunization Programme in a phased manner.
- Rubella vaccine is to be introduced as MR vaccine replacing the measles containing vaccine first dose (MCV1) at 9 months and second dose (MCV2) at 16–24 months.

FAQs

Q. What is the mode of administration of BCG vaccine?

Ans. MOA of BCG vaccine is intradermal.

Q. What is the site of administration of BCG vaccine?

Ans. SOA of BCG vaccine is on left arm just above the insertion of deltoid muscle.

Q. Why BCG is given in left arm?

Ans. BCG is given in deltoid area of left arm to differentiate it from smallpox vaccine scar which was conventionally given on right arm deltoid area. It also helps in assessing the vaccine status of the child during vaccination surveys done in future.

Q. Does BCG protect against adult type/pulmonary tuberculosis also?

Ans. No, BCG does *not* provide protection against adult type of tuberculosis. It only prevents severe form of childhood tuberculosis like TB meningitis and miliary Tb.

Q. What is dose of BCG vaccine?

Ans. In newborn it is 0.05 ml, while in post-neonatal period it is 0.1 ml.

Q. Which strain is utilized to prepare BCG vaccine?

Ans. WHO recommends "Danish 1331 strain" for the production of BCG vaccine. This strain is a sub-strain of the original Calmette strain of BCG. BCG laboratory at Guindy, Chennai, is using this strain for the production of BCG vaccine since 1967.

Q. Till what age can the pentavalent vaccine be given?

Ans. Under the Routine Immunization Programme of Government of India (GoI), pentavalent vaccine can be given to any child between the age of 6 weeks and 1 year.

Q. What are the side effects of pentavalent vaccine?

Ans. No serious side effects have been reported against pentavalent vaccines. However, local reactions such as pain and swelling at the site of vaccination and fever may be reported. These symptoms appear one day after vaccination and stay for 1–3 days.

Q. What are the important milestones of development of immunization in India?

Ans. The important milestones of development of immunization in India are listed in Table 5.2.

Table 5.2: Milestones of development of immunization in India

S.No.	Programme	Year
1.	Expanded Programme of Immunization (EPI) launched in India	1978
2.	Universal Immunization Programme (UIP)* started in 31 districts	1985
3.	UIP universalized to cover the entire country.	1990
4.	UIP became a part of Child Survival and Safe Motherhood (CSSM) Programme in the country.	1992
5.	First National Immunization Day for Polio eradication.	1995
6.	UIP became a part of Reproductive and Child Health (RCH) Programme in India.	1997
7.	UIP became part of overall umbrella health programme, National Rural Health Mission (NRHM) in India	2005
8.	Second dose of measles was included in the National Immunization Schedule New Initiatives	2010
9.	National Teeka Express	2013
10.	Four new vaccines have been introduced into the country's Universal Immunization Programme (UIP)	2014
11.	Mission Indradhanush by Government of India	2014
12.	"Babies Need You" by UNICEF	2015
13.	National Vaccine Reminder	2015

*Initially it was launched in 31 districts

Q. What are the contraindications of pentavalent vaccine?

Ans. Pentavalent vaccines are contraindicated in children having serious adverse reactions to the first dose of vaccine.

Note: Students are advised to remember the similar questions related to other vaccines also.

National Teeka Express

The National Teeka Express is an initiative by Government of India to protect children from life-threatening childhood diseases.

What was the need?

Under Routine Immunization Programme, ANM is responsible for offering the vaccines to children for which she has to collect the vaccines from storage point (cold chain point, i.e. PHC) and transport them to actual vaccination site for carrying out vaccination, but it was observed that ANMs have to collect the vaccines on the day preceding the immunization day, which may compromise the cold chain maintenance and lead to possible loss of potency of vaccine. Therefore increased chance of adverse events following immunization and risk of cold chain failure may be there.

For this reason, Government of India has launched the "Teeka Express". In this 'TE' designated vehicles under the brand name of 'National Teeka Express' will distribute the vaccines and complementary logistics from last cold chain point to immunization session sites. 'Teeka Express' will also be used with reverse cold chain to bring back the open and unused vaccines for use in subsequent sessions. It will also serve as a mobile healthcare delivery unit for the areas where there is no healthcare facility or health worker.

It will be piloted in 69 high priority districts with difficult areas and low immunization coverage. For these districts, 1,850 vehicles are planned to be procured with the assistance from Government of India.

Mission Indradhanush (MI)

The Mission Indradhanush was launched on birth anniversary of Bharat Ratna, Pandit Madan Mohan Malaviya ji and birthday of Bharat Ratna, Atal Bihari Vajpayee. The ultimate goal of MI is to achieve full immunization coverage for all children in India by 2020, thus protecting them against seven vaccine preventable childhood diseases.

This will be achieved by identifying 201 high focus districts in the country in the first phase which have nearly 50% of all unvaccinated or partially vaccinated children. These districts will be targeted by intensive efforts to improve the routine immunization coverage. 297 districts will be targeted for the second phase in the year 2015.

The focused and systematic immunization drive will be through a "catch-up" campaign mode where the aim will be to cover all the children who have been missed out for immunization. Under Mission Indradhanush, four special vaccination campaigns will be conducted between April and July 2015 with intensive planning and monitoring of these campaigns. Technical support to the Ministry will be provided by WHO, UNICEF, Rotary International and other donor partners. Mission Indradhanush will include other support mechanisms in the form of mass media, interpersonal communication, and sturdy mechanisms of monitoring and evaluation.

"Babies need you" by UNICEF

UNICEF, India launched "babies need you", a digital campaign that appeals to parents, future parents and the general public to put vaccination high on their priority list. The campaign will raise awareness about the need for full immunization for each and every child in the community and family. This initiative supports the efforts led by the Government of India for routine immunization under Mission Indradhanush.

As part of the "babies need you" campaign materials, UNICEF has developed three videos that challenge Indian parents to question their concerns regarding their children's health.

"National Vaccine Reminder" is another initiative by GoI, which will send reminders for every vaccination of the child through SMS, two days in advance. These reminders will continue till the child is 12 years old. The reminders will be sent after the child is registered through a SMS to 566778 in the following format: Immunize (space) child's name (space) child's date of birth. For example Immunize Sonu 01-01-15.

FAQs

Q. What is "Mission Indradhanush" and why was it started?

Ans. The Mission Indradhanush was launched on birth anniversary of Bharat Ratna, Pandit Madan Mohan Malaviya ji and birthday of Bharat Ratna, Atal Bihari Vajpayee. The ultimate goal of MI is to achieve full immunization coverage for all children in India by 2020, thus protecting them against seven vaccine preventable childhood diseases.

Q. Why it is called as "Mission Indradhanush"?

Ans. It is called "Mission Indradhanush" since the target is to cover 7 vaccine preventable diseases like the 7 colors in "Indradhanush". The seven vaccine preventable diseases are: 1. Tuberculosis, 2. Diphtheria, 3. Pertussis, 4. Tetanus, 5. Polio, 6. Measles, and 7. Hepatitis B.

Q. What is "National Teeka Express" and what were its objectives?

Ans. Under "National Teeka Express", vehicles will distribute the vaccines and complementary logistics from last cold chain point to immunization session sites, for proper maintenance of temperature till the last point in the cold chain, where the chances of failure of cold chain is maximum.

Q. Which agency had started "Babies need you" initiative?

Ans. UNICEF

Q. What does UNICEF stand for?

Ans. United Nation International Children's Relief Fund.

6

Planning an Immunization Session

Although there are certain activities to be carried out while planning and conducting an immunization session such as microplanning, preparing an area map, coordination between health workers such as ANM, AWW and ASHA, informing and motivating the beneficiaries, reporting and monitoring (mother child and tracking system); however, the students are primarily asked about method of estimation of doses for an immunization session in a subcenter. We will therefore discuss about the method of calculation of estimated doses in a subcenter.

Steps for calculation of estimated doses of vaccines in an immunization session at a subcenter area

1. Estimate the number of beneficiaries for vaccination, i.e. the number of pregnant women and infants: The annual and monthly targets. These numbers can either be estimated as discussed below or the accurate number of pregnant women and infants in an area is recorded on the basis of actual head count by the health worker (ASHA/AWW).

2. Accommodating for the wastage factor for each vaccine, calculate the doses of vaccine required.

3. Based on the number of doses/vaccine vial, calculate the number of vials required per month.

Method of estimation of the number of beneficiaries based on demographic indicators is discussed below:

For example, if the birth rate of the area is 30 per thousand live birth and IMR is 60 per thousand live birth in an area of 5000 population, then

- *Total number of live births/year*

  = Birth rate × Population of the area

  = 30/1000 × 5000 = 150/yr

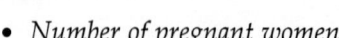

- *Number of pregnant women*
  = No of live births + 10% (for pregnancy wastage)
  = 150 + 15 = 165/yr
- *Number of infants alive at 1 yr*
  = *No. of live births – (IMR × No. of live births)*
  = 150 – (60/1000 × 150)
  = 141 (IMR being 60/1000)
- *Number of children below 3 yrs*
  = Approximately 8% of population
  = 8/100 × 5000
  = 400/yr
- *Number of children below 5 yrs*
  = Approx. 13% of population
  = 13/100 × 5000
  = 650/yr

Dividing the number of beneficiaries by 12, we get the number of beneficiaries per month.

Next, we calculate the beneficiaries for each antigen per month based on the number of doses required per beneficiary.

- TT = No. of pregnant women × 2
  Therefore for above example, the number of doses required would be 165 × 2 = 330

Similarly, for other vaccines

- BCG = No. of infants × 1 = 150
- OPV = No. of infants × 4 (include the birth dose for home deliveries) = 141 × 4 = 564
- DPT = No. of infants × 5 = 141 × 5 = 705
- Hep B = No. of infants × 3 = 141 × 3 = 423
- Measles = No. of infants × 2 = 141 × 2 = 282
- Vitamin A = No. of infants × 9 = 141 × 9 = 1269

Note: For calculation of **exact** no. of doses we have to also take wastage multiplication factor (WMF) into consideration, since there is wastage of 25% of the doses of vaccines during administration due to various reasons. The wastage multiplication factor is therefore 1.33 for almost all the vaccines. We, therefore multiply all the above calculated doses with 1.33 for obtaining the exact doses.

Note: Wastage multiplication factor for vitamin A and auto-disable syringes is 1.11

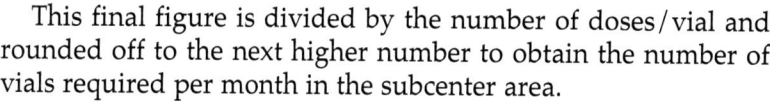

This final figure is divided by the number of doses/vial and rounded off to the next higher number to obtain the number of vials required per month in the subcenter area.

Note

- TT/BCG/DPT/Hep B vaccines vials contain 10 doses/vial
- OPV vial contains 20 doses/vial
- Measles vial contains 5 doses/vial.

For calculation of autodisable syringes and reconstitution syringes, we multiply the calculated requirement with a WMF of 1.11.

- 0.1 ml autodisable syringes (ADS) = (beneficiaries for BCG) × 1.11
- 0.5 ml ADS = (beneficiaries for TT + DPT + Hep B + measles) × 1.11
- *Reconstitution syringes* (BCG + measles vials) × 1.11

7

BCG Vaccine

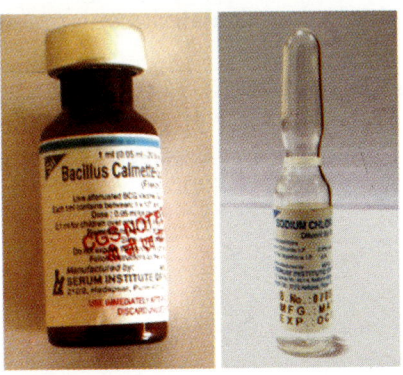

BCG vaccine (freeze dried) in amber colored vial and normal saline as diluent for reconstitution

Active Immunization

- *Type of vaccine:* Live attenuated, freeze dried bacterial vaccine.
- *Strains included in the vaccine:* Derived from bovine strain—Danish 1331 strain. It is produced in Guindy, India.
- *Contents*
  - 0.1–0.4 million live attenuated bacilli/dose.
  - It is stored in dark-colored bottle since it is light sensitive.
  - It has no preservative and therefore it should be used within 4 hours of reconstitution, otherwise there is a risk of toxic shock syndrome.
- *Diluent:* Normal saline.
- *Storage temperature:* 2–8°C
- *Age of administration:* Preferably at birth or within 14 days of birth; otherwise it should be given at the age of 6 wks along with other vaccines, i.e. DPT1, OPV1 and Hep B1.
- *Dose:* 0.05 ml before the age of 14 days and 0.1 ml after 1 month of age.

- *Route:* Intradermal (use a tuberculin syringe with 1 cm length, 26G/27G needle)
- *Site:* Left arm, just above the insertion of deltoid. If the injection is made too above, forward or backward, it may lead to axillary lymphadenitis.
- *Cleaning/preparation of site:* By sterile saline; no antiseptics to be used, since it may destroy the live attenuated bacterial component of the vaccine.
- *Phenomenon after vaccination:* Wheal of 5 ml at injection site, followed by papule (2–3 wks), ulceration (5–6 weeks) and scarring of 4–8 mm diameter (6–12 wks).
- *Contraindications*
  - Immunocompromised individuals especially those with deficient cellular immunity such as in hypogamma-globulinemia, leukemia, lymphoma, and HIV infection.
  - Patients on immunosuppressive treatment—corticosteroids, antimetabolites, and radiotherapy.
  - Patients suffering from generalized eczema, infective dermatoses, and pregnancy.
  - Gap of 4 wks is required between measles/MMR and BCG vaccine.
- **Effective mainly against** miliary and meningeal form of tuberculosis (75–86% efficacy). Less effective against pulmonary tuberculosis (50% efficacy). The duration of protection is about 15–20 years.
- *AEFI*
  - *Common minor vaccine reactions:* Local reaction (pain, swelling, and redness)
  - *Rare vaccine reactions*
    - Suppurative lymphadenitis (100–1000 per million dose)
    - BCG osteitis (0.01–300 per million dose)
    - Disseminated BCG infection (0.19–1.56 per million dose)
  - These reactions may occur within 1–12 months of administration of the vaccine.

FAQs

Q. Should BCG be administered to a child with asymptomatic HIV infection?

Ans. Global Advisory Committee on vaccine safety recommends that children known to be having HIV infection should not be immunized with BCG vaccine, even if they are asymptomatic, since the risk of developing disseminated BCG disease is increased in these children. The status of HIV infection in the first year of life should be assessed on the basis of direct demonstration of HIV virus, as the infants have "maternal antibody" which is transferred transplacentally.

Q. Can BCG be given along with OPV, DPT and hepatitis B?

Ans. BCG can safely be administered along with DPT and hepatitis B, but on different sites, without compromising the immune response to any of the antigens. BCG should not be given along with measles vaccine and a gap of at least 4 weeks should be kept in between the two vaccines since, measles vaccine is reported to decrease the cellular immunity, which may lead to tubercular infection, if BCG vaccine (which contains live attenuated bacteria) is administered.

Q. If a child could not be vaccinated with BCG vaccine at birth what should be done?

Ans. A child can be vaccinated within 14 days of birth with the BCG vaccine, else the child should be called at 6 weeks and administered BCG along with the first dose of DPT, OPV and Hep B, since a minimum interval of 4 weeks is to be maintained between two vaccines.

Q. Why is the dose of BCG vaccine before 14 days of age 0.05 ml, while that at 6 weeks is 0.1 ml?

Ans. Since BCG is administered intradermally, the space beneath the skin in neonates can accommodate only 0.05 ml of the vaccine; later the skin can accommodate 0.1 ml vaccine. If more than 0.05 ml is given in neonates, it may penetrate deeper causing lymphadenitis and local abscess formation or may ooze out through the puncture made in skin through the needle of the BCG syringe.

Remember: BCG is the only vaccine with a dose of 0.05 ml/0.1 ml; the rest of the vaccines are given in the dose of 0.5 ml.

Q. Is BCG vaccination an effective strategy for controlling tuberculosis?

Ans. Active case finding and treatment under DOTS is more effective in controlling tuberculosis than BCG vaccination. BCG vaccination is effective in preventing the childhood forms of tuberculosis, i.e. extrapulmonary and miliary tuberculosis. Its role in preventing pulmonary tuberculosis is questionable.

Q. Till what age can BCG be administered?

Ans. BCG can be administered till the age of 1 year in India. Beyond that age, it is not required, since the child acquires immunity through natural/subclinical infection.

Q. What should be done if the scar does not appear after administration of BCG vaccine?

Ans. Nothing is to be done. BCG should not be given again.

Q. What is the reason for local abscess formation after BCG vaccination and how should it be treated?

Ans. The local abscess formation may be due to subcutaneous injection of BCG or administration of another injection in the same arm within 6 months of administering BCG vaccine. The abscess should be aspirated if it does not heal on itself. If it still does not heal, it should be incised and local application of para-amino-salicylic (PAS) acid or isoniazid (INH) powder should be done daily.

Q. What are the recommendations regarding selective BCG vaccination in industrialized countries with low prevalence of tuberculosis?

Ans. Selective BCG vaccination is recommended in countries with an efficient notification system and with following criteria of "low endemicity":
  i. An average annual notification rate of smear positive pulmonary TB cases below 5/100,000
  ii. An average annual notification rate of tubercular meningitis in children aged under five years, below 1/10 million population during previous 5 years
  iii. An average annual risk of tuberculosis infection below 0.1%.

8

Diphtheria, Pertussis and Tetanus (DPT) Vaccine

Types of Immunizing Agents Available

1. **Combined/single vaccine**
2. **Antisera/immunoglobulin.**

Combined or mixed vaccines	Single vaccines
1. DTwP	1. FT (formal toxoid)
2. DtaP	2. APT (alum-precipitated toxoid)
3. DT	3. PTAP (purified toxoid aluminum phosphate)
4. Td	4. PTAH (purified toxoid aluminum hydroxide)
5. Tdap (adult type)	5. TAF (toxoid-antitoxin flocculus)

Contents of Different Types of Combined Vaccines

- *DTwP vaccine*
  - Diphtheria toxoid (20–30 Lf/dose)
  - Tetanus toxoid (5–25 Lf/dose)
  - Killed whole cell pertussis bacilli
  - Aluminum salt as adjuvant.
- *DTaP vaccine:* Acellular pertussis component reduces the minor adverse effects associated with whole cell pertussis (wP) component. The serious adverse effects are similar for both types. Also, the duration of protection against pertussis is shorter and no herd effect is documented with DTaP.

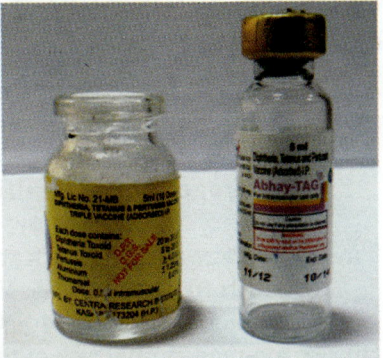

- *DT vaccine*
  - Same contents as DTwP/DTaP except for the absence of pertussis component.
  - It is recommended for children ≥7 years of age in whom pertussis vaccine is not indicated.
- *Td vaccine*
  - *Contents:* Usual dose of tetanus toxoid and only 2 units of diphtheria toxoid.
  - *Indication:* For children aged ≥7 years of age requiring immunization against diphtheria and tetanus only/in whom pertussis is contraindicated.
  - It is also indicated as replacement for TT in all situations where TT is given.
- *Tdap*
  - Those who have received the 3 doses of primary vaccination and 2 booster doses should be administered single dose of Tdap at the age of 10–12 yrs in deltoid.
  - Persons 7–10 yrs of age, who have not been fully immunized with all the doses of DTP: Give Tdap as the first dose and Td as subsequent doses if required.

Description of DPT Vaccine

- DPT Vaccine is of two types:
  - *Plain*
  - *Adsorbed:* Adsorption is usually done on the aluminum phosphate to increase the immunological effectiveness.
- *Storage temperature:* 2–8°C (should never be frozen)
- *Age of administration*
  - Primary vaccination: 6, 10, 14 weeks.
  - Boosters at 15–18 m and 5 years with DTwP and DTaP.
  - At 10–12 years of age: Single dose of Tdap in deltoid should be given to those who have received the 3 doses of primary vaccination and 2 booster doses.
  - Persons 7–10 yrs of age, who have not been fully immunized with all the doses of DTP: Give Tdap as the first dose and Td as subsequent doses if required.
- *Dose:* 5 doses; each dose is 0.5 ml
- *Route:* **DEEP** intramuscular because it causes intense local reaction and pain if injected superficially.

- *Site:* Anterolateral aspect of mid-thigh.
- *Catch-up schedule of vaccination* (catch up schedule means that the child has not been vaccinated at the age when he/she should be vaccinated. So now we are catching up with his immunization schedule!)
  - If last dose of DTP vaccine is given after 4 years of age, 2nd booster is not required.
  - Unimmunized child <7 years of age: DTwP/DTaP at 0, 1 and 6 m
  - Unimmunized child >7 years of age: Tdap, Td and Td at 0, 1 and 6 m.
- Immunization of children recovering from diphtheria, tetanus and pertussis is essential as natural disease does not offer complete protection.
- *Valid contraindications* (should not give the vaccine) for both DTwP and DTaP are:
  - Severe allergic reaction to previous doses
  - Encephalopathy
  - Progressive neurological deficit (relative contraindication).
- *Precautions (may or may not give the vaccine based on risk-benefit assessment)*
  - Persistent crying for >3 hrs
  - Fever >40.5°C
  - Hypotonic hyporesponsive episodes within 48 hrs of administration
  - Seizures with or without fever within 72 hrs of administration
- *Invalid contraindications* (conditions which *do not* require stopping of vaccination) of DPT are:
  - Temperature <40°C
  - Family history of seizures
  - Stable neurological conditions
- *Adverse effects*
  - *Local reaction:* Pain, swelling and redness at local site, fever, etc. reported in about 50% of doses.
  - *Rare vaccine reactions*
    - The severe adverse effects are very rare.

- They are considered to be the precautions or contra-indications for administration of subsequent doses of the vaccine.
- They are primarily due to the pertussis component of the vaccine.

The various rare vaccine reactions following DTwP administration are as follows:

- Fever >40.5°C
- persistent inconsolable crying for more than 3 hours occurs within 24 hrs of administration at a rate of <1/100 doses
- Seizures may occur within 3 days of administration at a rate of <1/100 doses
- Hypotonic hyporesponsive episodes may occur within 48 hours at a rate of 1–2/1000 doses
- Encephalopathy may occur with 2 days at a rate of $0–1/10^6$ doses
- Anaphylaxis is reported within 1 hour in $20/10^6$ doses.
- **Effectiveness** against diphtheria/tetanus after 3 doses: >95%.
- **Efficacy** of wP alone: 61–89%; efficacy of combination DTwP ranges from 46 to 92%.
- Severity of pertussis infection decreases with age, the pertussis component in DPT vaccine is not usually recommended after the age of 6 years.
- For immunizing children over 12 years of age and adults, the preparation of choice is dT, which is an adult-type of diphtheria tetanus vaccine.

For passive immunization: Antisera (prepared from horse serum) is given.

- *Dose:* 500–1,000 IU of diphtheria antitoxin
- *Route:* IM
- *Indications:* To susceptible contacts immediately following exposure
- *Duration of protection:* 2–3 weeks

FAQs

Q. What should be the route of administration of DPT vaccine?

Ans. All vaccines containing adjuvants should be injected as DEEP intramuscular injection, otherwise the local reactions such as pain at the injection site might be more severe.

Q. What is the frequency of adverse reactions due to DPT?

Ans. Fever and local reactions such as pain, swelling and redness occur at a frequency of 50%. The frequency of rare vaccine reactions is as follows:

- Seizures and persistent (>3 hrs) inconsolable crying and screaming <1%
- Hypotonic, hyporesponsive episodes: 0.1–0.2%
- *Anaphylaxis:* 20 per lakh doses
- *Encephalopathy:* 1 per lakh doses

Q. What are the most severe complications following DPT vaccination?

Ans. The most severe complications following DPT vaccination are primarily due to the pertussis component and are mainly neurological which include convulsions, encephalopathy/ encephalitis, infantile spasms and Reye's syndrome. The risk of such complications is rare (1: 170000 doses).

Q. What are the contraindications for DPT vaccine?

Ans. Minor illnesses (fever, cough, etc.) are not a contraindication to DPT vaccination. In case of serious illness or hospitalized children, it should not be given. Also, DPT should *not* be administered if the child has had severe reactions (collapse, shock, persistent screaming, high fever >40°C, neurological complications, convulsions or anaphylactic reactions) to a previous dose of DPT. Convulsions occurring within 72 hours and encephalopathy occurring within 7 days of vaccination are attributed to vaccination.

Q. What is the vaccine efficiency after three doses of DPT vaccination?

Ans. The vaccine efficiency after the three primary doses of DPT vaccination is 70%.

Q. Why is the first dose of DPT vaccine given so early at the age of 6 weeks?

Ans. Since the adult females of childbearing age do not have sufficient levels of antibodies against diphtheria and pertussis since these antigens are not well-tolerated in adults, these antibodies are not transferred to the child during pregnancy. The child is therefore susceptible to both diphtheria and pertussis right from the birth. The Global Advisory Group of the Expanded Programme on Immunization therefore recommends the administration of DPT as early as 6 weeks after birth for early protection against the diseases.

Q. What should be the time interval between two doses of DPT vaccine?

Ans. Ideally the interval between two primary doses of DPT vaccine should be 8 weeks but to increase the compliance to vaccination schedule and reduce the drop-out rate, an interval of 4 weeks between two primary doses is advised. The level of final immunity after the three doses by both the schedules (interval of 8 weeks/4 weeks) is comparable.

Q. What is the site of vaccination of DPT?

Ans. In children especially infants, DPT is given on the anterolateral aspect of mid-thigh which is a safe area as it has less of nerves and vessels and also has adequate muscle mass as compared to the gluteal region which has sciatic nerve which can be damaged. Also, gluteal region has more fat and less muscle mass which inhibits the absorption of the vaccine and thus leads to inappropriate immune response.

Q. What are the directions that should be given to the parents after DPT vaccination?

Ans. Parents should be told that the vaccination causes some local reactions such as pain and fever. Following instructions should be given:

- The site of vaccination should not be rubbed vigorously
- Cold compress should be applied at the site of vaccination. The induration and pain at the site of vaccination usually subsides in 2–3 days. In case it persists for more than three days and is accompanied by fever, we should suspect abscess formation or cellulitis and appropriate antibiotics should then be administered.

- Paracetamol should be given to child in case of fever.
- In case of any serious reactions such as convulsions, etc. the parents should report immediately to the doctor.

Q. Are there any indication of giving reduced dose (<0.5 ml) of DPT?

Ans. There are no indications of reducing the dose of DPT vaccine. Not even in preterms or malnourished children, since lower dose will not produce optimum immune response.

Q. What should be done if the DPT vaccine is frozen?

Ans. The vaccine should be discarded as ALL T series vaccine are freeze sensitive and lose their potency on freezing and thawing. The DPT vaccine should never be frozen.

Q. If a child does not develop fever following DPT vaccination, does it imply that the vaccine was not potent?

Ans. Development of fever and pain is a "Reaction" of the body to vaccine and its incidence is about 50% of doses and therefore does not happen in every child. It does not imply that the vaccine is not potent.

Q. Can DPT be given to children having nonprogressive neurological disorder such as cerebral palsy?

Ans. Yes DPT can safely be administered to children with cerebral palsy since it is a nonprogressive neurological disorder. Only progressive neurological disorders such as encephalitis, encephalopathy, infantile spasms, etc. are contraindications for DPT vaccination.

Q. What is the difference between DTwP and DTaP vaccine?

Ans. The diphtheria and tetanus components of both the vaccines are same; however, the pertussis component varies in both the vaccines.

The DTwP contains whole cell of killed pertussis bacilli, whereas the DtaP contains acellular killed pertussis bacilli. The contents of both the vaccines are as follows:

- *DTwP vaccine*
  - Diphtheria toxoid (20–30 Lf/dose)
  - Tetanus toxoid (5–25 Lf/dose)

- Killed whole cell pertussis bacilli
- Aluminum salt as adjuvant
- *DTaP vaccine:* Acellular pertussis component reduces the minor adverse effects associated with whole cell pertussis (wP) component. However, the duration of protection against pertussis is shorter and no herd effect is documented with DtaP. The serious adverse effects are similar for both types.

Q. If a child receives all the three primary doses of DPT at scheduled intervals and another child receives the three doses at irregular intervals such as at 3, 6 and 9 months, what will be the difference in the immunity status of these two children?

Ans. The final immune status of both the children will be comparable, however, the child having irregular vaccination schedule will be susceptible to infections of diphtheria and pertussis till all the three primary doses have been received, i.e. till 9 months of age; whereas the child completing the vaccination at 14 weeks will acquire immunity early and will therefore be protected against infections early in life.

Q. A child has recovered from diphtheria. Does he require the vaccine?

Ans. The immune response after the natural disease is variable, therefore the child should be vaccinated irrespective of the previous disease status, so that he acquires sufficient and reliable immunity against the disease.

In people with no vaccination, protective level of immunity is reported to have been developed in response to inapparent skin infections with C. diphtheria in approximately 75% children by the age of 6–8 years. However, in younger children it is safe and advisable to vaccinate the children for timely protection from the disease which is maximum between the age of 1 and 5 years of age.

Q. Does immunization prevent against the carrier state of diphtheria?

Ans. Immunization affords protection against the disease but does not prevent the carrier state, since the vaccine being a toxoid is

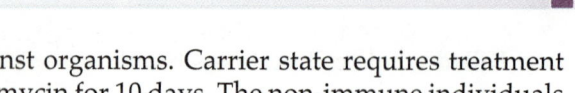

not directed against organisms. Carrier state requires treatment with oral erythromycin for 10 days. The non-immune individuals do not get protection by the high levels of population immunity.

Q. What is the role of vaccination in "Contacts" of diphtheria cases?

Ans. The management of contacts varies according to their previous vaccination status:

If the child has received primary dose or booster dose:

- *Within last two years:* Nothing is required to be done
- *>2 years ago:* A booster dose of diphtheria toxoid is to be given
- *Non-immunized close contacts:*
  - Give prophylactic penicillin/erythromycin
  - Diphtheria antitoxin (1000–2000 units)
  - Diphtheria toxoid first dose
  - Daily surveillance for clinical signs of diphtheria for 1 week following exposure.

Q. Which type of vaccine should be used to immunize children >12 years of age against diphtheria, pertussis and tetanus? What is the schedule of vaccination in adults?

Ans. The vaccine of choice for immunizing children >12 years of age is dT, which contains the usual content of tetanus toxoid (5–25 Lf) but contains a lesser amount of diphtheria toxoid (2 Lf) as compared to the usual amount of 25 Lf in the DPT or DT vaccine preparation. Also, it does not have the pertussis component since the risk of having pertussis after 6 years of age is minimal whereas the risk of neurological side effects increases.

Schedule of dT vaccination: Two doses at 4–8 weeks interval; booster after 6–12 months.

Q. Can DPT be given along with measles vaccine?

Ans. Yes, DPT can safely be given along with measles vaccine since DPT vaccine contains toxoids and killed bacilli, which do not have the potential to cause the disease. Only live attenuated vaccines like BCG are contraindicated with measles vaccine as they may lead to a disease state.

Q. Can DPT vaccine be given after an episode of measles in a child?

Ans. Yes, DPT vaccine can be safely administered in a child recovering from measles, since DPT has toxoids and killed bacilli, which do not have the potential of causing a disease. Also DPT vaccine evokes a humoral immune response; whereas measles infection leads to a cell-mediated immune response.

Q. Can DPT be given along with BCG vaccine?

Ans. Yes, DPT can safely be given along with BCG vaccine. In fact, a child who has not received BCG vaccine at birth or within 14 days of birth, is administered BCG vaccine along with the first dose of DPT at 6 weeks of age. Almost all the vaccines can be given with DPT. Only precaution that has to be kept in mind is that the site of vaccination should be different for all the vaccines.

9

Tetanus Vaccine

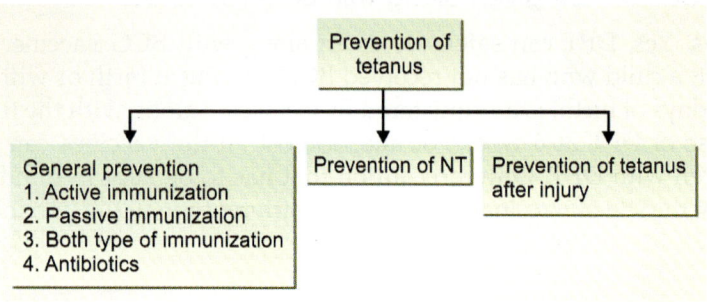

Prevention of tetanus
→ General prevention
1. Active immunization
2. Passive immunization
3. Both type of immunization
4. Antibiotics
→ Prevention of NT
→ Prevention of tetanus after injury

I. Active Immunization

Preparations available for active immunization include:

1. ***Combined vaccine:*** DPT (already discussed under DPT): Administered at 6, 10, 14 weeks, booster at 18 m and 5–6 years. Subsequent booster of TT every 10 yrs.

2. *Monovalent vaccines*
   - *Plain or fluid (formal toxoid):* Provides rapid protection
   - *Tetanus toxoid (adsorbed):* Provides higher and longer lasting immune response.

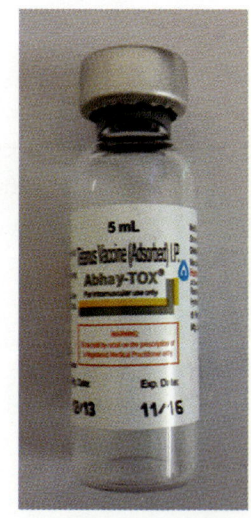

Tetanus Toxoid, Adsorbed

- ***Contents:*** 5 Lf of toxoid.
- ***Storage temperature:*** 2–8°C. It is one of the most heat stable vaccine
- ***Route:*** Intramuscular (IM)
- ***Site:*** A / L aspect of mid-thigh in children and deltoid in adults.
- ***Dose:*** 0.5 ml

- *Schedule:* 2 doses at 1–2 months interval, 1st booster after 1 year and third booster after 5 years.
- If booster doses are administered more frequently than indicated, it leads to increased frequency and severity of local and systemic reactions.
- *Contraindications:* None
- *Adverse effects:* Mild, local pain and tenderness.
- *Efficacy:* Approximately 100%

II. Passive Immunization

- *Human tetanus hyperimmunoglobulin* (produced by serum institute of India, Pune)
  - *Dose:* 250–500 IU
  - Protection up to 30 days
- *Horse ATS:* Dose is 1500 IU subcutaneous after sensitivity testing
  - Protection for 7–10 days
  - Causes sensitivity reactions, especially to the second and subsequent doses.
  - Leads to production of antibodies to the ATS. Therefore subsequent doses of ATS become ineffective.

III. Active and Passive Immunization

- Requires administration of both antisera and the toxoid.
- Human tetanus hyperimmunoglobulin (250–500 IU) or Horse ATS (1500 IU) in one arm for passive immunization and 0.5 ml adsorbed TT in another arm for active immunization.
- Followed by 0.5 ml TT after 6 wks
- 3rd dose of TT one yr later

PREVENTION OF NT

- Well controlled through clean delivery practices which are effective in prevention of neonatal tetanus.
- Includes practicing the 5 cleans during delivery—clean surface, clean hands, clean cut, clean tie and clean cord, i.e. no application on the stump of the umbilical cord.
- In unimmunized pregnant women, 2 doses of TT s/b given
  - *1st dose* should be administered as early as possible
  - *2nd dose:* A month later and at least 2–3 wks before delivery.

- In subsequent pregnancies that occur in next 5 years, one dose of TT would suffice.
- If there is a gap of more than 5 years from previous TT vaccination, 2 doses of TT would again be needed.
- In partially immunized pregnant women with:
  - *3 primary doses:* 2 doses during first pregnancy and one dose in second pregnancy
  - *3 primary doses and one booster dose:* One dose each, in both first and second pregnancy.
  - *3 primary doses and two booster doses:* One dose only in first pregnancy. No further doses required in subsequent pregnancy.
- In fully immunized women with 3 primary doses, two boosters in childhood and one Tdap in adolescence: No further doses are required.
- In areas with high incidence of NT the primary 2 dose course is given to all women of child bearing age.
- Infants born to unimmunized mothers should be given antitoxin 750 IU within 6 hrs of birth (Table 9.1).

	Table 9.1: Prevention of tetanus after injury	
	Surgical toilet in all wounds: Cleaning, removal of dead tissue, thorough washing to prevent anaerobic environment.	
	Wounds <6 hrs, clean, non-penetrating with negligible damage	*Other wounds*
Immunity category	*Treatment*	*Immunity category and treatment*
A	Nothing more required	Nothing more required
B	Toxoid 1 dose	Toxoid 1 dose
C	Toxoid 1 dose	Toxoid 1 dose + Human Tet Ig
D	Toxoid complete course	Toxoid complete course + Human Tet Ig

A—Those who have completed the full course of tetanus toxoid within past 5 years
B—Those who have completed the full course of tetanus toxoid >5 years but <10 years ago
C—Those who have completed the full course of tetanus toxoid >10 years ago
D—Those who have not completed the full course of tetanus toxoid or in whom the immunization status is unknown

Remember, the treatment and immunization is same in both clean and dirty wound for all the categories except in the last two categories, which also requires immunoglobulin for immediate protection.

FAQs

Q. For how long is the child of an immunized mother protected against tetanus infection?

Ans. The child of an immunized mother is protected for a period of less than 6 months by the transfer of passive immunity to the child. Therefore the primary immunization by DPT should be provided at the scheduled age of 6, 10 and 14 weeks for effectively protection against all the three diseases.

Q. If an individual has recovered from tetanus, does he still need to be vaccinated?

Ans. An individual who has recovered from tetanus still needs to be vaccinated since the amount of toxin responsible for causing the disease do not produce sufficient levels of protective immunity.

Q. Does Tetanus vaccination/infection provide herd immunity?

Ans. Tetanus vaccination/infection does *not* provide *herd immunity*. Therefore for effective prevention all individuals at risk should be vaccinated.

Q. Is it important to administer tetanus toxoid after every injury?

Ans. The administration of TT depends on the previous vaccination status of the individual and the condition of the injury.

All wounds should undergo surgical toilet which includes cleaning of the wound, removal of dead tissue and thorough washing to prevent anaerobic environment. Active and passive immunization should be undertaken on the basis of previous immunization status and the type of wound are given in Table 9.2:

Table 9.2: Active and passive immunization in case of any injury for prevention of tetanus

Previous immunization status		Treatment for			
		Wounds <6 hrs, clean, non-penetrating with negligible damage		Other wounds	
		Toxoid	Human Tet Ig	Toxoid	Human Tet Ig
Those who have completed the full course of tetanus toxoid	Within past 5 years	No	No	No	No
	>5 years but <10 years ago	Yes (1 dose)	No	Yes (1 dose)	No
	>10 years ago	Yes (1 dose)	No	Yes (1 dose)	**Yes**
Not completed TT vaccination/unknown immunization status		Yes (complete course)	No	Yes (complete course)	**Yes**

If the wound is clean, no immunoglobulin is required. Immunoglobulin is required in **only contaminated wounds** and if the time since completion of TT vaccination is more than 10 years.

Q. If a 7-year-old completely vaccinated child is brought to your clinic with a dirty wound, which vaccines should be given to him for prevention of tetanus?

Ans. Neither active nor passive vaccination is required to be given to the child since he had completed the full course of tetanus toxoid within last 5 years. However, the wound should be cleaned thoroughly and dirty tissue should be removed. He should also be given penicillin/erthromycin to combat the vegetative forms of *Clostridium tetani*.

Q. What is the effect of giving frequent doses of TT?

Ans. Frequent doses of TT administration may lead to hyperimmunization and increased side effects. This is important for females who might be vaccinated in every pregnancy and the duration between two pregnancies is less than 5 years.

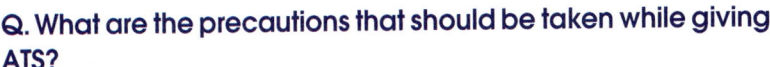

Q. What are the precautions that should be taken while giving ATS?

Ans. ATS may cause a generalized anaphylaxis because it is prepared from horse's serum, which is foreign to the human body. To counter the effects of the same, we should keep the following medicines ready:

- *Adrenaline solution 1 in 1000:* 0.5–1 ml IM
- *Hydrocortisone 100 mg:* IV injection

   Also a test dose of ATS (0.1 ml) should be given *subcutaneously* (not intradermally) and the patient should be observed carefully for any local or systemic reactions such as fall in pulse rate/ blood pressure, shock, dyspnea, etc. If there is a reaction, the rest of the ATS should be given in gradually increasing fractions after treatment with adrenaline. If the reactions persist, ATS should not be given.

Q. What are the other adjuncts to the treatment of a wound for prevention of tetanus?

Ans. Passive immunization by ATS provides immediate protection but has its side effects. Tetanus toxoid does not provide immediate protection. Antibiotics such as penicillin or erythromycin are effective against the vegetative forms of *Clostridium tetani* but are ineffective against spores. Also, antibiotics are effective only when given within 6 hrs of injury. However, it is not certain whether the antibiotic will reach the bacilli especially if there is a dead tissue in the wound. Antibiotics are an adjunct to vaccination, not a substitute.

Q. After how much time of administration of tetanus toxoid does the immunity develop?

Ans. A minimum of 2 weeks is required for development of antibodies after active immunization with tetanus toxoid. Therefore, if there is a need for immediate protection such as in case of an injury in unvaccinated child or an elective or emergency surgery, the child may be afforded protection by passive immunization, i.e. ATS/human tetanus immuno-globulin.

Q. Can active and passive immunization against tetanus be carried out simultaneously?

Ans. Yes, both tetanus toxoid and ATS/human tetanus Immunoglobulin may be given simultaneously but they should be given on separate arms/sites and by separate syringes.

Q. What are the adverse reactions following tetanus vaccination?

Ans. Common minor vaccine reactions following tetanus toxoid immunization include local reaction such as pain, swelling and redness (10%) and malaise and non-specific symptoms at the rate of 25%. The rare reactions include brachial neuritis ($5-10/10^6$ cases) within 2–28 days and anaphylaxis ($1-6/10^6$ cases) with an onset within one hour of administration of vaccine.

10

Measles Vaccine

Active Immunization

- *Type of vaccine:* Live attenuated, freeze dried.
- *Strain used:* Edmonston Zagreb strain grown on human diploid cells or purified chick embryo cells.
- *Contents of the vaccine*
  - Each 0.5 ml of the vaccine contains 1000 $CCID_{50}$ of measles virus
  - Sorbitol and hydrolized gelatin are added as stabilizer, and small amount of neomycin.
  - No preservatives (thiomersal) are added in measles vaccine. Therefore reconstituted vaccine looses its potency after 1 hr at 37°C; and after 6 hrs at 2–8°C.
- *Diluent:* Distilled water.
- *Storage:* Can be frozen or stored at 2–8°C
- Heat labile and light sensitive vaccine. Therefore supplied in amber colored vial.
- *Age:* 1st dose at 9 m; 2nd dose at 1.5 yrs under NIS.
- *Dose:* 0.5 ml (≥1000 viral infective units)
- *Route and site:* Subcutaneous, right arm
- *Reactions*
  - Local reaction (pain, swelling and redness) at a rate of 10%
  - Irritability, malaise and nonspecific symptoms, fever (5%)
  - Rash
  - Febrile seizures (in 6–12 days; frequency: 3/1000 doses)
  - Anaphylaxis if allergic to egg (with vaccines produced on chick embryo cells)

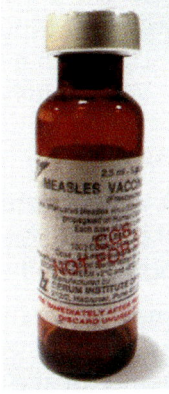

- *A very severe side effect:* **Toxic shock syndrome (TSS)** can occur if the vaccine gets contaminated or it is used beyond 1 hr of reconstitution at 37°C and 6 hrs at 2–8°C. Toxic shock syndrome is characterized by watery diarrhea, vomiting, high fever within a few hours of immunization. The case fatality rate of TSS is high. It often leads to death within 24–48 hours and is an indicator of programme error. The management consists of early recognition and prompt treatment in hospital by antibiotics and fluids.
- No person to person transmission of vaccine strain has been reported
- *Immunity:* Develops 11–12 days after vaccination
- At 9 m—90% seroconversion
- At 11–12 m: 99% seroconversion
- *Contacts* can be protected if vaccine is given within 3 days of exposure since the incubation period of vaccine induced measles is 7 days as compared to 10 days for naturally acquired measles.
- *C/I:* Pregnancy, acute illness, deficient CMI, high fever , allergy to vaccine contents intake of steroids and immunosuppressants. Early stage of HIV infection is not a contraindication.
- *Immune response:* Both cellular and humoral
- Can cause a depression of cell mediated immunity. However, it can be given to those with early HIV infection or latent/unrecognized tuberculosis.
- Can be given with all childhood vaccines except BCG.

Immunoglobulin
- Effective if administered early in incubation period within 3-4 days of exposure
- *Dose:* 0.25 ml/kg body weight
- Vaccine to be given after 8–12 weeks.

FAQs

Q. Why is measles vaccine recommended to be administered at completion of 9 months of age only? Can we give it earlier than 9 months?

Ans. Measles is recommended specifically at 9 months of age group because maternal antibodies persist in infants up to 7–8 months of age which interfere with the vaccine antigen.

We can offer the vaccine before 9 months of age under following conditions:

a. During an epidemic

b. Whatsoever the reason may be, if mother says that she cannot return back at 9 months of age for vaccination, then we can offer the vaccine even at 5–6 months of age.

c. If child has come in a contact with a case of measles.

Q. What changes have recently been made in NIS with respect to measles vaccine?

Ans. GOI has recently approved the introduction of 2nd dose of measles vaccine in the routine immunization schedule which will be offered at 16–24 months of age.

Q. At what age of administration does measles vaccine show highest seroconversion rate? If it differs from 9 months what is the reason?

Ans. The highest seroconversion rate of measles vaccine is observed at 11–12 months of age therefore ideally the vaccine should be administered at 11–12 months of age but still the first dose of vaccine is offered at 9 months because the maternal antibodies remain in the infant up to 7–8 months of age. There is a possibility that these antibodies may persist for a bit longer and interfere with the measles vaccine given at 9 m of age. Therefore to avoid this interference due to maternal antibodies, it is best to immunize the child at 11–12 m for best seroconversion rates. However, if the age of administration of first dose of measles is postponed till 11 to 12 m, most of the infants with waning maternal antibodies will become susceptible and may contract the disease. Therefore on assessing the risk-benefit it has been decided to immunize the child at 9 months with first dose and give a second dose at 16–24 m for those who have not seroconverted with the previous dose and boost the effect of the previous dose in those who have seroconverted.

Q. Can we offer measles vaccine to an adult?

Ans. Yes, measles vaccine can be offered to adults provided that they have not received the vaccine during childhood and also have not suffered from an attack of measles disease.

Q. What is TSS? How it is related with measles?

Ans. Toxic shock syndrome (TSS) is a severe and preventable side effect of measles vaccine as well as BCG vaccine which is characterized by fever, diarrhea, vomiting, blood in stools, Disseminated intravascular coagulation (DIC), shock and ultimately death within 24–48 hours if not treated promptly. It occurs due to contamination of the reconstituted measles vaccine. The contamination is usually caused by staphylococcal toxin. It can be prevented by proper storage of vaccine and also vaccine should be used immediately after reconstitution. It is an indicator of programme error.

Q. A 4-month-old child has come in contact with the case of measles, is it necessary to give measles vaccination to the child?

Ans. No, since the child remains protected till 5–6 months of age because of the maternal antibodies.

Q. Measles vaccine should be kept in which part of ILR?

Ans. Measles vaccine should be stored in the bottom part of the ILR just above the OPV while in the refrigerator it should be kept in uppermost portion or in chiller tray.

Q. What precautions should be undertaken while mixing the diluents in measles vaccine?

Ans. Distilled water is used to reconstitute the vaccine. The temperature of the diluent should be same as that of the vaccine. Only diluents supplied along with the vaccine should be used for reconstitution. The reconstituted vaccine should be used within 4 hours of reconstitution and any leftover vaccine should be discarded after that.

Q. Is it required to shake the vaccine vigorously after reconstitution?

Ans. No, shaking the vaccine vigorously can lead to frothing and bubbles formation which can lead to difficulty in actual estimation of the dose of measles vaccine.

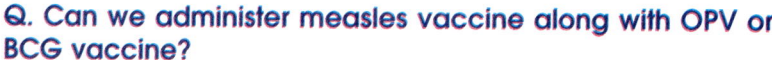
Q. Can we administer measles vaccine along with OPV or BCG vaccine?

Ans. We can offer the measles vaccine with OPV but BCG vaccine should not be offered along with measles vaccine since measles vaccine can interfere with immunity, especially T cell-mediated immunity for 4–6 weeks which can reduce the successful uptake of BCG vaccine or may lead to tuberculosis infection.

Q. Is there any harm if measles vaccine is given intramuscularly?

Ans. If measles is given intramuscularly no harm will occur, but it should preferably be given subcutaneously.

Q. Can the vaccine cause measles?

Ans. Since measles vaccine is live, it can cause measles-like symptoms, however, it does not cause measles disease.

Q. Does appearance of measles like symptoms after measles vaccine indicate effective development of immunity as compared to those who do not develop it?

Ans. No, measles-like symptoms after measles vaccine only indicates adverse reactions of the vaccine. It is not an indicator of development of immunity.

Q. If we have applied spirit on the site of injection before injecting the measles vaccine what precaution should we take?

Ans. Spirit should be allowed to evaporate completely before vaccine is administered, so that it does not inactivate the live attenuated components of the vaccine.

Q. Why is neomycin added in the measles vaccine?

Ans. Neomycin helps in preventing the bacterial contamination of the vaccine.

Q. What is the strategy for measles elimination and rubella control?

Ans. Measles elimination and rubella control strategy includes:

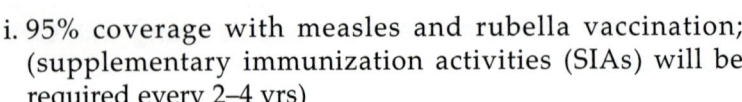

i. 95% coverage with measles and rubella vaccination; (supplementary immunization activities (SIAs) will be required every 2–4 yrs)
ii. Case-based surveillance with adequate laboratory support
iii. Prevention of outbreaks
iv. Linkages with other child health interventions (vitamin A administration in high risk areas)
v. Increased public confidence and demand for immunization

Q. What is the vaccination strategy for measles elimination?

Ans. Vaccination strategy for measles elimination includes catch up, keep up and follow-up.

- *Catchup*
  - One time nationwide vaccination campaign
  - 9 months–14 yrs regardless of vaccination/ds status
- *Keep up*
  - Routine vaccination >95% for each successive birth cohort
- *Follow-up*
  - Subsequent nationwide campaign every 2–4 yrs targeting all children born after the catchup campaign

India recently completed a measles immunization campaign targeting 139 million children aged 6 months to 10 years in 14 states.

Introduced a second dose of measles immunization through routine immunization in another 21 states.

11

Rubella Vaccine

- *Type of vaccine:* Live attenuated viral vaccine
- *Strain used:* RA-27/3 produced in human diploid fibroblast. It prevents subclinical infection with wild virus.
- *Storage:* Freeze dried form; can be frozen or stored at 2–8°C
- Light sensitive, heat sensitive, should be used within 6 hours of reconstitution.
- *Age of administration:* After one year of age.
- *Dose:* 0.5 ml
- *Route:* Subcutaneous
- *Immunity:* Lifelong
- *Contraindications:* Pregnancy, immunocompromised persons
- *Adverse effects:* Mild rash, arthralgia, arthritis, thrombocytopenic purpura.

FAQs

Q. What is the vaccination strategy for control of congenital rubella syndrome (CRS)?

Ans. Vaccination strategy for control of congenital rubella syndrome (CRS) includes the following steps in a sequential manner:

Vaccination of women of 15–34/39 years of age →all children 1–14 yrs of age →all children at 1 yr of age →routine universal immunization at 1 year of age.

Measles elimination is an opportunity for rubella elimination. Rubella is less infectious than measles. If countries use combined measles-rubella vaccine, then when measles is eliminated, rubella and CRS will also be eliminated. Rubella vaccine is highly effective (95% with one dose), safe (whether given singly or in combination) and affordable.

Q. Why rubella vaccine is given on a priority basis to women of reproductive age group?

Ans. Rubella vaccine is given on priority basis to women of reproductive age group since the prime objective of giving rubella vaccine is to prevent the CRS (congenital rubella syndrome) as it is a serious diseases and if a child develops CRS he will suffer with the defects for the rest of his/her life. Therefore as a priority group, women of reproductive age group are targeted for rubella vaccination. However, it is contraindicated among pregnant women.

Q. As mentioned in the answer to above question that rubella vaccine is contraindicated in pregnancy but can be offered to women of reproductive age group, after how long a woman is advised to conceive?

Ans. Once a woman has received the rubella/MMR vaccine, she is advised to conceive after a minimum of 3 months period.

12

Mumps Vaccine

- *Type of vaccine:* Live attenuated freeze dried viral vaccine.
- *Vaccine strains used:* Jeryl Lynn, Leningrad-3, L-Zagreb, Urabe AM9 strain and RIT 4385.
- *Formulations available:* Available as monovalent vaccine containing only mumps virus or in combination with other vaccine viruses such as measles, rubella and varicella (MM, MMR, MMRV)
- *Storage:* S/b frozen for long-term storage. Can be stored at 2–8°C.
- Light and heat sensitive. Should be used within 4-6 hrs after reconstitution.
- *Dose:* 0.5 ml; 2 doses are required for durable protection. First dose in children over 1 year of age at 12–15 m and second dose at 4–6 years of age.
- *Route:* Subcutaneously.
- Can be given along with all other childhood vaccines except BCG.
- *Contraindications:* Pregnancy, immunocompromised state, severe illness.
- Now recommended for routine immunization for children over 1 year of age in the form of MMR.
- *Adverse effects:* Fever, febrile seizures, aseptic meningitis (Jeryl Lynn strain has the lowest rate), transient parotitis, thrombo-cytopenia. There are no long-term sequelae associated with mumps vaccination.

FAQs

Q. Which strain of mumps vaccine should not be used in national immunization programmes and why?

Ans. WHO recommends that Rubini strain should not be used due to its lower effectiveness.

Q. A child has developed parotitis after MMR vaccine, is it due to MMR vaccine?

Ans. Yes, it is most likely due to side effect of mumps component of the MMR vaccine.

Q. Is it safe to offer MMR vaccine to a breastfed child?

Ans. Yes. Breastfeeding does not interfere with the response to MMR vaccine.

Q. What are the strategies for achieving mumps elimination?

Ans. For achieving mumps elimination, following strategies have to be undertaken:
1. Very high coverage with first dose of mumps vaccine.
2. High coverage of 2nd dose.
3. Catchup immunization of subsequent susceptible cohorts.

13

Poliomyelitis Vaccine

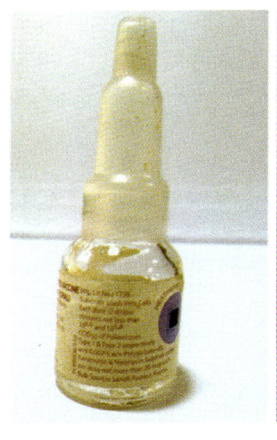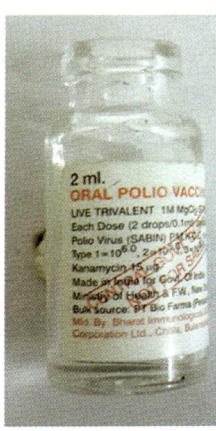

There are two types of vaccine available for immunization against polio. The differences between the two vaccines are listed in Table 13.1.

Table 13.1: Differences between killed and live poliovirus vaccine		
Characteristics	*Killed IPV (Salk)*	*Live (Sabin)*
Type	Killed formalized virus	Live attenuated virus
Strain used	40, 8, 32 D Ag of Type 1, 2 and 3	3, 1, 3 L TCID$_{50}$
Dose	0.5 ml	2 drops
Administration	Subcutaneous/ IM	Oral
Schedule	4 doses. First 3 doses at a gap of 1–2 m and 4th dose after 6–12 m. 100% effective after 2nd dose. Revaccination every 5 years till 18 yrs of age.	5 doses in clinic and 3 doses in community

Contd...

Table 13.1: Differences between killed and live poliovirus vaccine (*Contd.*)

Characteristics	Killed IPV (Salk)	Live (Sabin)
Immunity	Humoral, not rapid	Local and humoral, rapid
Prevents	Paralysis; not reinfection	Paralysis and reinfection
Control of epidemic	Not useful. May precipitate paralysis	Useful
Manufacture	Difficult	Easy
Cost	More	Cheap
Storage and transport	Does not require stringent condition, but should be refrigerated to maintain potency. Should *not* be frozen.	Require stringent condition
VAPP	Not reported	1 in 2.4–3.3 million
Protection	Only vaccinated individual	Contact immunity
Immuno-compromised state	Safe	Not advised
In pregnancy and old age	Safe	Not advised
Adverse reactions	Minor: Local erythema (0.5–1%), induration (3–11%) and tenderness (14–29%)	VAPP

Some Other Important Points about IPV

- *IPV has 3 strains:* Type 1: Mahoney; Type 2: MEF-1; Type 3: Saukett
- IPV may contain trace amounts of formaldehyde, streptomycin, neomycin or polymyxin B.
- Some versions may contain preservative phenoxyethanol (0.5%)
- Thiomersal (incompatible with IPV antigenicity) and adjuvants are not used.
- Combined vaccine (with diphtheria, tetanus, whole-cell or acellular pertussis, Hep B, Hib) is also available. In combined vaccine, pertussis vaccine or the alum has an adjuvant effect.
- Recent OPV are heat stabilized by adding $MgCl_2$. Can be stored at 4°C for 1 yr; 25°C: 1 month

What is sequential administration of IPV and OPV?

- Sequential administration is defined as 1–2 doses of IPV followed by ≥2 doses of OPV.
- *Advantage:* Reduces or prevents VAPP with maintenance of high level of intestinal mucosal immunity.

Strategy in Areas with Compromised OPV Efficacy

- Monovalent OPV_1 (mOPV1) SIAs for interrupting wild poliovirus type 1 (WPV1) transmission.
- Periodic bivalent OPV (bOPV) SIAs to maintain immunity against WPV3.
- After interruption of WPV1, mOPV3 SIAs to interrupt WPV3 transmission with periodic bOPV SIAs to maintain immunity against WPV1.
- 2 tOPV SIAs per year to maintain immunity against type 2 poliovirus.

Vaccine Derived Poliovirus

- OPV can lead to vaccine associated paralytic polio (VAPP), which are clinically indistinguishable from polio caused by WPV but can be distinguished by lab diagnosis.
- The incidence of VAPP has been estimated to be 4/1,000,000 individuals per year in countries using OPV. It can occur in both the recipients and their unimmunized contacts.
- Most frequently associated with Sabin 3 (60%) followed by 2 and 1.
- Detection is done by real time reverse transcriptase polymerase chain reaction.

FAQs

Q. What are the objectives of Polio Eradication and Endgame Strategic Plan 2013-2018

Ans. The objectives of the plan are as follows:

1. Detect and interrupt all poliovirus transmission by continued and enhanced surveillance
2. Strengthen immunization system and withdraw oral polio vaccine for elimination of risk due to vaccine derived poliovirus.

3. Containment and certification of the eradication of wild polio virus from all WHO regions by 2018.

4. Legacy planning by transfer of learning, assets and infrastructure from Polio Programme to other relevant programmes.

Q. When will the use of OPV be discontinued?

Ans. OPV will be replaced with IPV once all wild poliovirus transmission has been interrupted all over the world.

Q. A child has suffered from polio. Does he still need to be vaccinated?

Ans. Immunity following infection with WPV is fairly reliable. However, there is NO cross immunity and therefore infection with one serotype does not provide protection against other serotypes and reinfection can therefore occur. It is, therefore, imperative to vaccinate the child by OPV/IPV even after he/she has suffered from polio.

Q. Is a newborn child protected against polio infection?

Ans. If the mother is immune to polio, maternal antibodies are transferred to the fetus but the immunity wanes off gradually during the first 6 months of life. The child should therefore receive the first dose of vaccine at 6 weeks of life and complete the schedule by 14 weeks for effective protection against the disease.

Q. What instructions regarding feeding are to be given to the parents of children receiving OPV?

Ans. The children should not be given hot water, hot milk or hot fluids for half an hour after the administration of the vaccine. However, breastfeeding is not contraindicated and can be done whenever the child is hungry.

Q. A child is having diarrhea. Should he be administered OPV?

Ans. Diarrhea is not a contraindication to OPV. However, the dose should not be counted and the child should be revaccinated as soon as he/she recovers from the diarrheal episode.

Q. What are the contraindications of OPV?

Ans. Since OPV is a live attenuated vaccine, it is contraindicated in immunocompromised states such as leukemia, malignancy, pregnancy and children on corticosteroids or having acute illness such as hepatitis.

Q. Is there any Immunoglobulin available for preventing polio?

Ans. Normal human immunoglobulin is available and is protective for a few weeks. It provides protection against paralytic polio but does not prevent subclinical infection. Also it is effective only if given shortly before infection. It is ineffective after development of clinical symptoms. The dose is 0.25–0.30 ml per kg body weight. The vaccine should be given at least 4 weeks after the immunoglobulin. In practice, the immunoglobulin is rarely used due to the widespread use of vaccines.

Q. Usually, the live attenuated vaccines require single dose; but OPV requires multiple doses. What is the reason for the same?

Ans. There are several reasons for the same:
- The vaccine is given orally, therefore there are chances for the vaccine loss through GI tract. The whole vaccine may not be taken up as compared to other vaccines given through parenteral route.
- OPV is a polyvalent vaccine and therefore it takes time for development of immunity against each serotype individually. It has been reported that one serotype gains foothold at one time. After multiple doses (six), the immunity against all the three serotypes is achieved in the range of 82–95%.
- OPV requires stringent temperature control. Therefore, the vaccine may lose potency and may become ineffective. Giving multiple doses ensures that it is taken up by the body on one or the other occasion.
- For these same reasons, some of the individuals who have received the vaccine still might develop the disease.

Q. What is the need of having gut immunity for protection against polio?

Ans. Gut immunity is provided by OPV which does not allow the wild poliovirus to gain a foothold in the intestine and thereby prevents infection especially during epidemics.

Q. Which immunity is better—gut immunity or systemic immunity?

Ans. A good level of systemic immunity is better than only gut immunity. If the child has both gut immunity and systemic immunity, he will be prevented from polio infection. Systemic immunity can be achieved from both IPV and OPV, whereas gut immunity is provided by only OPV. IPV is reported to provide higher systemic immunity than OPV.

Q. If there is a polio epidemic in an area, what steps should be undertaken?

Ans. In the event of an epidemic, oral polio vaccine should be administered to all the children under five years of age irrespective of their immunization status. Also, continuous surveillance for the cases of acute flaccid paralysis should be done and the isolation of virus strain from the stool sample must be done. Apart from this, no injectables should be given and surgical operations such as tonsillectomy should be deferred till the cessation of the epidemic, as they may precipitate the paralysis. In addition to these, people should be educated to maintain food, water and personal hygiene to prevent the feco-oral transmission of the polio infection.

Q. What is the mechanism of increased risk of paralysis due to polio, if an injection is administered or a surgery is performed during a polio epidemic?

Ans. No injectables should be given and surgical operations such as tonsillectomy should be deferred till the cessation of the epidemic, as they may precipitate the paralysis. This increased risk of paralysis is due to the fact that the inflammation around the surgical or injection site elicits a vascular response in the corresponding segment of the spinal cord. This, in turn, leads to migration of poliovirus along the axons to the anterior horn cells.

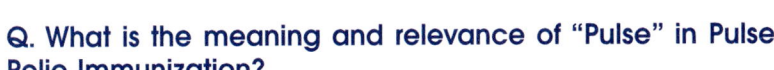

Q. What is the meaning and relevance of "Pulse" in Pulse Polio Immunization?

Ans. Pulse means intermittent and simultaneous administration of OPV to all the susceptible children (<5 years of age) irrespective of their previous immunization status. By this, the vaccine virus replaces the wild virus from the community since all the susceptible children are vaccinated. Pulse Polio Programme is supplemented by the routine immunization.

Q. What happens if a child is given more than two drops of OPV?

Ans. Nothing except mild diarrhea can occur on higher doses. However, the directions regarding the dose should be adhered to.

Q. What is VAPP?

Ans. Vaccine associated paralytic polio (VAPP) is polio occurring due to vaccine virus. It is a rare adverse event (4 cases per 1,000,000 birth cohort per year). It can occur in the vaccinated individuals as well as their unimmunized contacts. It is postulated that attenuated poliovirus, on repeated passages through unimmunized individuals converts into a wild virus thus causing paralysis due to polio. Serotype 3 is most commonly associated with this adverse event (60% cases). VAPP cannot be differentiated from paralytic polio due to wild virus clinically. It requires virological methods for their identification and classification.

Q. What are the points in favour/against the use of IPV?

Ans. With the achievement of goal of eradication of polio from India, it is time now to shift to IPV administration which provides good protection against the infection to an individual. Also the risk of VAPP is absent and it does not requires stringent storage temperature.

The drawbacks are that it requires expertise in administration of IM injections, but that can be done by the health workers effeciently. Also the herd effect provided by the OPV is no longer required after achieving the eradication of polio.

Under National Immunization Schedule IPV is being included along with the third dose of DPT, along with the regular OPV vaccination.

Q. Can OPV be given to a preterm baby?

Ans. OPV can be given to a preterm baby but not while he/she is in nursery since infection with OPV virus can lead to VAPP in susceptible neonates by cross infection.

Q. How many boosters of OPV are required under NIS?

Ans. Under NIS, there are 4 primary doses: OPV—0, 1, 2 and 3 at birth, 6, 10 and 14 weeks and a booster at 16–24 months along with DPT booster.

Q. If an unvaccinated child of 18 months reports for vaccination, how many doses of OPV should be given to him?

Ans. Three primary doses at an interval of 1 month and a booster dose after 6–12 months may be given to the child.

Q. A child has suffered from poliomyelitis. Does he still require vaccination with OPV?

Ans. Poliovirus has three serotypes. Infection with one serotype does not provide immunity against other serotypes. Therefore even if a child has been infected, he/she should be given the vaccine for development of immunity against other serotypes. The vaccine should be administered after at least 4–8 weeks of the attack of poliomyelitis.

Q. Is administration of polio vaccine during prodromal phase of poliomyelitis preventive against polio?

Ans. Polio vaccine will not prevent paralytic polio if administered during prodromal or preparalytic stage of polio.

Q. What should be done if a child regurgitates or vomits within one hour of OPV administration?

Ans. OPV should be given again.

Q. If a child has measles/chickenpox, should he be given OPV?

Ans. A child with measles can be given OPV after about a month of the attack of measles/chickenpox.

Q. What are the recommendations for temperature maintenance regarding OPV?

Ans. Following are the recommendations for polio vaccine storage:

- For storage for long duration (till 1 year), OPV should be stored at −20°C in deep freezer.
- At PHC, it is kept at +2 to +8°C (1 month) in ILR.
- During immunization session: In ice packs and VVM should be checked before vaccination.
- In refrigerator, it should be kept just below the freezing compartment.

14

Viral Hepatitis

HEPATITIS A

Passive Immunization

By human immunoglobulin:
- *Indication:* Those who are at higher risk.
- *Dose:* 0.02 ml/kg (1–2 m)/ 0.06 ml/kg (3–5 m)
- *Effectiveness:* 80–90% effective (if given within 14 days of exposure). Protective within hours
- *Disadvantage*
  - Cost
  - Limited duration of protection (3–5 m)
  - Since vaccines are equally effective and lead to rapid production of antibodies, use of immunoglobulins is decreasing.

Active Immunization

Two types of vaccines are available—killed and live attenuated.

Live vaccine is produced in China and available in some countries, while killed is most commonly used worldwide. The differences between the two types of vaccines are listed in Table 14.1:

Table 14.1: Differences between killed and live attenuated hepatitis A vaccine

Characteristics	Killed vaccine	Live attenuated vaccine
Vaccine strain	Formaldehyde inactivated, HM 175/GBM strain; aluminum hydroxide as adjuvant	H2 or LA-1 HAV strain
Vaccine efficacy	90–100%	95–100%
Injection route	Intramuscular	Subcutaneous/IM

Contd...

Table 14.1: Differences between killed and live attenuated hepatitis A vaccine (*Contd...*)

Characteristics	Killed vaccine	Live attenuated vaccine
Schedule	1st dose: 12–18 months 2nd dose: 2 to 3 years	1st dose ≥12 months 2nd dose: After 6–18 m
Protection	Till 45 years Effective in outbreaks	3–15 years 100% efficacy in pre-exposure prophylaxis and 95% in post-exposure; not effective in outbreaks
Adverse effect	Local pain and swelling	-
Contraindications	Allergy to vaccine contents	Immunocompromised individuals
Protection gained	2–4 wks after 1st dose	
Booster	None recommended	
Dosage	0.5 ml (1–15 y); 1 ml in adults	
Injection site	Anterolateral aspect of thigh in children/deltoid in adults	
Storage	2–8°C	

FAQs

Q. Which other vaccines can be offered along with the hepatitis A vaccine?

Ans. Hepatitis A vaccine can be offered along with vaccines like hepatitis B, diphtheria, poliovirus (oral and inactivated), tetanus, oral and intramuscular typhoid, cholera, Japanese encephalitis, rabies, and yellow fever vaccines.

Q. Can we give immunoglobulin of hepatitis A simultaneously along with hepatitis A vaccine?

Ans. Yes, but at different anatomical sites.

Q. Is it advisable to offer hepatitis A vaccine before travel?

Ans. Yes, if the person is travelling to an area endemic for hepatitis A.

Q. How many days before travel should the first dose of hepatitis A vaccine be given to travelers visiting endemic areas of hepatitis A?

Ans. Ideally hepatitis vaccine should be administered at least 2 weeks before the journey for optimal immune response. However, Advisory Committee on Immunization Practices (ACIP) recommends that one dose of single-antigen hepatitis A vaccine administered at any time before departure may provide adequate protection for most healthy persons. However, older adults, immunocompromised persons and people with chronic liver diseases starting their journey within 2 weeks should receive both vaccine and Ig (0.02 ml/kg) simultaneously at separate anatomical injection sites for immediate protection.

Q. Is it safe to offer the hepatitis A vaccine during pregnancy?

Ans. Since the vaccine is inactivated therefore theoretically it can be safely administered among pregnant women. However, the safety of hepatitis A vaccination during pregnancy has not been proven till date.

Q. Is it safe to offer the hepatitis A vaccine among immunocompromised persons?

Ans. Yes.

HEPATITIS B (SERUM HEPATITIS) VACCINE

Active Immunization

Type of vaccine: Killed vaccine containing hepatitis B surface antigen

Formulations

- Monovalent
- Combination (with other vaccines like DPT, HiB, hepatitis A, etc.)
  Can also be classified on the basis of production process as:
- Plasma derived
- Recombinant type of vaccine. (Nowadays recombinant vaccine has replaced the plasma derived vaccine.)

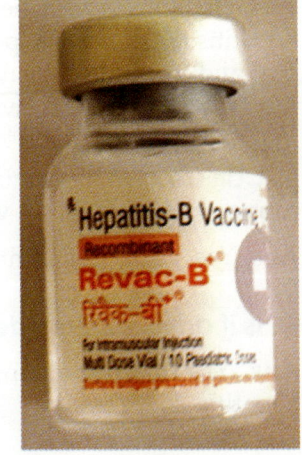

Characteristics of Plasma Derived Vaccine

- Formalin inactivated
- 1 ml contains 20 μg surface Ag
- *Route:* Intramuscular
- *Doses:* 3 doses (0, 1, 6 months); Booster at 3 yrs
- *Antibody response:* 95%

Characteristics of RDNA Yeast Derived

- Safe, effective and more cost effective
- Alum and lipid A are used as adjuvant in vaccine administered to patient with renal insufficiency
- *Route and site:* Deep IM. For greatest reliability of absorption of vaccine in adults, the deltoid muscle is preferred for injection as gluteal injection often results in deposition of vaccine in fat rather than the muscle, with reduced seroconversion. For infants and children, vaccine is offered in anterolateral aspect of mid-thigh
- *Storage:* At 2–8°C
- *Age of administration:* Can be offered at any age group
- *Dose*
  - Among children in India 4 doses of 0.5 ml are offered, one at the time of birth and rest along with three doses of DPT, i.e. on 6, 10 and 14 weeks. At birth only monovalent Hep B vaccine should be used
  - Among adults 1 ml each of three doses on 0, 1 and 6 months (each ml of vaccine contains 20 μg of HBsAg)
  - *In Type III countries:* 1st dose s/b given within 24 hours.
- *C/I:* Allergy to vaccine contents
- *Reactions*—very safe vaccine
- *Immunity:* Antibodies are produced in 95% of infants and children, if course of vaccine is completed but if primary vaccination is started in late age seroconversion rate of vaccine drops. The duration of protection is at least 15 years and for probably lifelong
- Contacts can be protected by offering the vaccine as early as possible along with the antibodies
- *Vaccine nonresponse:* <5% of person fail to develop immunity even after the administration the required number of vaccine doses

- Interruption of the vaccination schedule does not require restarting of the vaccine series. Instead the 2nd dose should be given as soon as possible and 2nd and 3rd dose separated by a minimum interval of 4 weeks.

Passive Immunization: Hepatitis B Immunoglobulin (HBIg)

- *Indications*
  - Surgeons/lab workers
  - Newborn infants of carrier mothers
  - Sexual contacts
  - Patients requiring protection after liver transplantation
- Should be given as soon as possible preferably within 6 hrs.
- Simultaneously draw blood for HBsAg.
  - If –ve for HBsAg: Start vaccination immediately
  - If +ve for anti-HBs: No further action is needed
- *Dose:* 0.05–0.07 ml/kg between 2 doses, 30 days apart

Active and Passive Immunization

Simultaneous administration of HBIg and hepatitis B vaccine is more efficacious than HBIg alone.

FAQs

Q. Which vaccine is preferred, plasma derived or recombinant vaccine and why?

Ans. Recombinant vaccine is preferred over plasma derived vaccine as it is cost effective, purified and more immunogenic. Moreover, the plasma derived vaccine has risk of transmitting the infections like HIV/AIDS, etc.

Q. If a person has received the first dose of hepatitis B vaccine from one manufacturer, can he receive the other doses from different manufacturer?

Ans. Yes. No differences in immune response are observed when vaccines from different manufacturers are used to complete the vaccine series.

Q. What will happen if the doses of hepatitis B vaccine have been interuppted? Does the vaccine series require to be restarted?

Ans. No, as is true for all other vaccines, the series does not need to be restarted. If the vaccine series was interrupted after the first dose, the second dose should be administered as soon as possible. The second and third doses should be separated by an interval of at least 8 weeks. If only the third dose is delayed, it should be administered as soon as possible.

Q. What will happen if hepatitis B vaccine has been administered concurrently with other vaccines?

Ans. Since hepatitis B vaccine is a very safe vaccine, it can be offered at the same time with other vaccines. No interference with the antibody response of the other vaccines has been demonstrated. In fact, it is being administered along with DPT, OPV and sometimes BCG under the NIS. Separate body sites and syringes should be used for simultaneous administration of different vaccines.

Q. How long does protection from hepatitis B vaccine last?

Ans. The protection will last for at least 15 years and with recent scientific evidence it is reported to last lifelong. Cellular immunity appears to persist even though antibody levels might become low or decline below detectable levels.

Q. Why should an infant receive hepatitis B vaccine at birth before hospital discharge, even if the mother is negative for hepatitis B surface antigen (HBsAg)?

Ans. Both, hepatitis B vaccine and hepatitis B immunoglobulin (HBIg) are given to infants born to HBV-infected mothers within 12 hours of birth, to protect them from perinatal infection. However, the hepatitis B infection status of all the mothers is not known due to various reasons such as errors or delays in documentation, testing and reporting, therefore administration of the first dose of hepatitis B vaccine soon after birth to all infants provides protection to all of them against perinatal infection, if it occurs. It also increases the child's likelihood of completing the vaccine series on schedule.

Q. Is hepatitis B vaccine contraindicated during pregnancy or lactation?

Ans. No. Hepatitis B vaccine is a killed vaccine and also a very safe vaccine, therefore neither pregnancy nor lactation is a contraindication for the vaccine.

Q. Can hepatitis B vaccine be given to immunocompromised persons, such as persons on hemodialysis or persons with HIV infection?

Ans. Yes, although a larger vaccine dose is required to induce protective antibody in hemodialysis patients.

Q. What will happen if vaccine is offered to a person who has been infected with HBV?

Ans. Persons who have already been infected with HBV will receive no benefit from vaccination.

Q. What is current recommendation for the booster doses of hepatitis B vaccine?

Ans. A booster dose should be administered when anti-HBs levels decline to <10 mIU/ml. Persons with normal immune status who have been completely vaccinated, do not require booster doses. Booster doses are recommended only in certain circumstances: Patients on hemodialysis, immunocompromised persons (e.g. HIV-infected persons, hematopoietic stem-cell transplant recipients, etc.).

Prevention of Hepatitis C

- No vaccines available
- Prevention by avoiding infected blood and body fluids

Prevention of Hepatitis D

- Vaccination with HBV
- Carriers of HBV are not protected by vaccination

Prevention of hepatitis E (enterically transmitted hepatitis non-A and non-B)

- Personal and community hygiene similar to Hep A.
- No vaccine/Ig available

15

Chickenpox Vaccine

Passive Immunization

- Chickenpox may be prevented or modified by varicella-zoster immune globulin (VZIg).
- *Indications:* High risk groups including
- Immunocompromised individuals
- Susceptible pregnant women exposed to varicella, and
- Neonates born to mothers who developed varicella 5 days before to 2 days after delivery.
- Has no preventive value in established disease.
- *Dose:* 12.5 IU/kg body weight up to a max of 625 units.
- *Route:* Intramuscular injection.
- *Doses and schedule:* Administered as soon as possible after exposure (within 96 hours); 2 doses, 3 weeks apart
- Should not be given along with vaccine

Active Immunization

- *Type of vaccine:* A live attenuated, freeze dried vaccine based on the Oka strain (developed by Takahashi et al in Japan) has been available since 1974.
- *Storage:* During transport, maintain the vaccine at a temperature between –58°F and +5°F (–50°C and 15°C). May be stored at refrigerator temperature (36°F to 46°F, 2°C to 8°C) for up to 72 continuous hours prior to reconstitution. Vaccine stored at 2°C to 8°C which is not used within 72 hours of removal from +5°F (15°C) storage should be discarded.
- Reconstituted vaccine should be discarded, if it is not used within 30 minutes.
- *Immune response:* Induces both humoral and cellular immunity.

- *Dose*
  - *For children from 1 year–13 years:* 0.5 ml SC single dose/ two doses, 6 weeks or 3 months apart.
  - *For those >13 years of age:* 2 doses must be given, 4–8 weeks apart.
- A single dose achieves over 95% seroconversion.
- *Age of administration:* The vaccine must be given after one year of age.
- *Route:* Subcutaneous
- Vaccine can be used among HIV infected children including those who are on ARV therapy.
- HIV testing is not a prerequisite for varicella vaccination.
- *Contraindications* and precautions include:
  - Pregnancy, allergy to neomycin, immunodeficient state, malignancy, steroids administration and recent administration of blood, plasma, or immune globulin.
  - Salicylates are avoided for 6 weeks after giving this vaccine to prevent Reye's syndrome.
- *Risk factors for vaccine failure and breakthrough varicella*
  - Age at vaccination (<15 m)
  - Receipt of steroids
  - Administration of vaccine within 28 days of MMR vaccine

WHO's Position on Active Immunization

- WHO recognizes that in most developing countries, other VPDs cause greater morbidity and mortality.
- As a consequence, varicella vaccine is not a high priority for routine introduction into national immunization programmes.
- The WHO recommends that "routine" childhood immunization against varicella may be considered in countries where:
- This disease is a relatively important public health and socioeconomic problem,
- The vaccine is affordable, and
- High (85–90%) and sustained vaccine coverage can be achieved.

FAQs

Q. What are the rare vaccine reactions that can occur with varicella immunization?

Ans. Febrile seizures at a rate of 4–9/10,000 doses can occur after varicella immunization. The risk of seizures depends on age and the risk is lower in infants under four months of age. The treatment consists of supportive care which includes paracetamol and cooling for febrile seizure. Anticonvulsants are rarely required.

Q. Is the vaccine effective in preventing chickenpox after exposure?

Ans. The vaccine has no role in prevention after the onset of disease. However, VZ immunoglobulin is effective in preventing the disease if administered within three days of exposure to chickenpox. It may also modify the severity of the disease.

Q. What is the duration of protection provided by the vaccine?

Ans. According to current evidence, it is reported that the vaccine induced protection lasts for a period of 10 years on an average. This duration of protection depends on the boosting effect due to the wild varicella-zoster virus infections. Boosters after 4–6 years would increase the duration of protection significantly but are not recommended at present in individuals <13 years of age.

Q. What is the effectiveness of vaccine?

Ans. Vaccine effectiveness against moderate or severe disease has been reported to be 97%. If varicella occurs after vaccination, it is mild in nature.

Q. What is the storage temperature of varicella vaccine?

Ans. The vaccine should be kept away from light and stored at 2–8°C (see above the text).

Q. What are the adverse effects that may follow varicella vaccination?

Ans. Fever and local reactions at the injection site may occur. Vesicular rash may occur about three weeks following vaccination at the injection site or may be generalized. This vesicular rash may be infectious and may transmit the infection through contact of vesicular fluid only; *not* through respiratory route or through papules. To prevent the transmission of infection the vesicles should be covered, handwashing should be encouraged and separation of vaccinated individual from immunocompromised individuals and schools, etc. should be done till the lesions have crusted.

Q. Is it necessary to vaccinate every child against chickenpox?

Ans. The WHO recommends that routine childhood immunization against varicella may be considered in countries where:
- This disease is a relatively important public health and socioeconomic problem,
- The vaccine is affordable, and
- High (85–90%) and sustained vaccine coverage can be achieved.

In India, it is an optional vaccine and not included under National Immunization Schedule. Although the mortality rate due to chickenpox is less, but it may cause complications such as pneumonia in children and is an important cause for sickness absenteeism in schools. Moreover, an immunized person has been reported to have milder disease than unimmunized individual.

Q. What is a chickenpox party?

Ans. There is a concept of a chickenpox party in developed countries in which children are taken to a party in the house of a child suffering with chickenpox, so that other children can also develop chickenpox. As we all know that chickenpox is a mild disease in childhood and its severity increases several times in those having a disease for the first time in adulthood. So parents prefer to have their children suffer from chickenpox in childhood so that they are immune for the rest of their life.

Q. If chickenpox infection can lead to development of immunity for the rest of the life, why do we vaccinate the children? Why do not we allow them to contract chickenpox infection?

Ans. It is true that "disease acquired natural immunity" is better than "vaccine acquired immunity", but it is not without a cost.

The disease causes suffering and complications which might be fatal at times. It is also not sure that every child will contract the disease in childhood, so waiting for the disease to happen is not wise.

Q. In whom is the chickenpox vaccine contraindicated?

Ans. Chickenpox vaccine is contraindicated in the following conditions/individuals with:
- Severe life-threatening allergy to gelatin and neomycin
- Active infection with fever
- Pregnancy (females should not get pregnant for 3 months following vaccination)
- Immunocompromised individuals: Cancer, lymphoma, etc.
- On corticosteroids/immunosuppressive drugs.

Q. If a child has been exposed to a case of chickenpox what should be done?

Ans. If the child has been vaccinated earlier or has had chickenpox earlier, nothing needs to be done. A nonvaccinated child or one who has not had the disease earlier should be given the Ig as soon as possible (preferably within 3 days of exposure). The vaccination will reduce the seriousness of the disease if infected.

16

Meningococcal Meningitis Vaccine

Types of Vaccine

Two types of vaccines are available against *Neisseria meningitidis*
1. *Polysaccharide vaccines:* Short duration of protection
2. *Polysaccharide-protein conjugate vaccines:* Better herd immunity and increased immunogenicity in children <2 yrs.

Characteristics of Polysaccharide Vaccines

- *Formulations*
  - Bivalent (serotypes A, C),
  - Trivalent (serotypes A, C, W135),
  - Quadrivalent (serotypes A, C, W135, Y)
- *Content:* 50 μg of each of the individual polysaccharides
- *Dose:* Single dose, 0.5 ml
- *Age of administration:* ≥2 yrs; revaccination after 3–5 yrs in high-risk groups.
- *Route:* Subcutaneously/IM
- *Adverse reactions:* Mild, pain and redness at injection site, transient fever.
- *Immunity:* Protection within 7–10 days of vaccination
- *Storage:* 2–8°C

Conjugate Vaccines

- *Formulations*
  - Monovalent (A/C), alum (adjuvant) and thiomersal (preservative), conjugated to 10–33 μg of tetanus toxoid
  - Quadrivalent (4 μg each of A, C, Y and W135 polysaccharide conjugated to 48 μg of diphtheria toxoid)
  - *Combination:* Hib and *Neisseria meningitidis* group C (Hib Men C)

- *Route:* IM (deltoid / anterolateral aspect of mid-thigh in children <12 months)
- *Dose:* 0.5 ml
  - Monovalent A: Single dose (1–29 yrs)
  - Monovalent C
    - *≥12 months children, teenagers and adults:* Single dose
    - *Children 2–11 months:* 2 doses at 2 months interval and booster about 1 yr thereafter.
    - *Quadrivalent:* Single dose (≥2 yrs)
- *Storage:* 2–8°C
- *Indications of vaccination:* Routine vaccination is undertaken in certain high-risk groups such as:
  - Terminal complement component deficiencies
  - Anatomic or functional asplenia
  - Laboratory personnel and healthcare workers exposed routinely to *Neisseria meningitidis*
  - Persons with HIV infection
  - In close contacts of patients with meningococcal disease.
- Single dose of polysaccharide vaccine is recommended for travelers above 18 months of age going to high-risk area.
- Revaccination may be indicated for persons at high-risk for infection (living in endemic areas) particularly for children who were first vaccinated when they were less than four years of age
- *Safety:* Safe in pregnancy

FAQs

Q. What are the common adverse effects of the meningococcal vaccine?

Ans. Meningococcal vaccine causes only mild local reactions such as redness and pain at the injection site in about 71% vaccines and fever in some which lasts for 1–2 days. Paracetamol is effective in controlling fever. Brief fainting spells are also reported in adolescents. These can be prevented by sitting or lying down for 15 minutes after vaccination. Severe allergic reactions are rare.

Q. After how many days following vaccination does the immunity develop?

Ans. Immunity develops within 7–10 days following vaccination and remains effective for approximately 3–5 years.

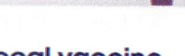

Q. Against which serogroups is the meningococcal vaccine effective?

Ans. Meningococcal vaccine is effective against four serogroups: A, C, W135 and Y. There are various options available such as monovalent, bivalent, trivalent and quadrivalent vaccines. They are also available as combination vaccines along with Hib vaccine.

Q. To whom is meningococcal vaccine given on a priority basis?

Ans. The most common age group at which an individual is vaccinated is ≥2 years as a single dose.

Monovalent Men A conjugate vaccine is given to individuals 1–29 years of age as single dose.

Men C vaccine is offered to children aged ≥12 months, teenagers and adults.

Children 2–11 months need 2 doses at an interval of 2 months and a booster after 1 year of the second dose.

Q. What is the route of administration of meningococcal vaccine?

Ans. Polysaccharide vaccine is administered subcutaneously whereas conjugate vaccines are given intramuscularly.

Q. Will a child be totally protected against meningitis after he/she is vaccinated with meningococcal vaccine?

Ans. There are several serotypes of *N. meningitidis* which cause meningitis. The vaccines do not provide cross immunity and are effective against the strain that is present in the vaccine. So a child may not be totally protected against meningitis after vaccination. However, the vaccines provide immunity against the common serogroups—A, C, W135 and Y. Parents should be vigilant for the signs and symptoms of meningitis and should consult the doctor as soon as possible since effective antibiotics (penicillin, ceftriaxone and 3rd generation cephalosporins) can save the lives of 95% of patients if started within 2 days of illness.

Q. Can the meningococcal vaccine actually cause meningitis?

Ans. No, the vaccines cannot cause meningitis since they are polysaccharide and conjugate vaccines; *not* live attenuated vaccines.

Q. What is the status of natural immunity in an individual against meningitis?

Ans. Children in younger age group are more susceptible than the older persons, since the older individuals acquire natural immunity through subclinical disease (most commonly), clinical disease or vaccination. Passive immunity is transferred from the mother to newborn child, yet the highest attack rate is found in infants 3–12 months of age.

Q. If a person has had meningitis and is still surviving, does this mean he/she is immune?

Ans. As stated above, having clinical disease provides immunity against the disease; however, since there are various serotypes of the bacteria, it is possible that the person may have been infected with one serotype for the first time and consequently developed immunity against that serotype only. He may develop the infection from another serotype later.

Q. Which group of people are at increased risk of meningococcal infection and should therefore be immunized?

Ans. Following group of individuals are at an increased risk of meningococcal infection and should therefore be immunized:
- Children and adolescents
- People/students living in dormitories or overcrowded conditions
- People travelling to endemic areas such as Africa
- Military recruits
- Laboratory personnel exposed to the meningococcal bacteria
- Individuals with asplenia and complement component deficiency conditions.

Q. Which individuals should not be vaccinated?

Ans. Vaccine should not be given under following conditions:
- Allergy to a previous dose or a component of the vaccine
- Individuals with any other acute/severe illness should be vaccinated after their recovery.

17

Influenza Virus Vaccine

Influenza virus undergoes frequent mutations due to antigenic shifts and drift phenomenon. Vaccines are effective against the specific strain of the virus against which they were manufactured and are therefore ineffective against other strains. The vaccine composition is therefore changed periodically (twice in a year) to match with the prevalent/expected strains.

Characteristics of Vaccine

- Recommended in selected population groups:
  - In industry to reduce absenteeisms
  - Public servants: Police, fire protection, transport and medical care.
  - Persons with underlying chronic disease and their contacts
- HIV patient can be safely vaccinated
- Highly effective (70–90%)
- Vaccine must be administered at least 2 weeks before the onset of the epidemic.

Characteristics of Killed/Inactivated Vaccine

- May contain inactivated whole virus, split product or subunit surface antigen (Ha or Na).
- *Content:* 15 μg of Ha of both H1N1 and H3N2 and one influenza B strain.
- *Dose and route:* A single inoculation of 0.5 ml (adults and children >3 yrs) or 0.25 ml (6 months–3 years) subcutaneously/ IM.
- In children <9 years: 2 doses, 1 month apart may be given.
- Minimum age of administration: 6 months
- *Efficacy:* 70–90%

- *Duration of effectiveness:* 6–12 months. Ab increase in 1 wk and reach max in 2 wks
- Revaccination is required annually
- *Time of vaccination:* Just before the onset of rainy season.
- *Side effects:* Fever, pain, GBS (rarely), allergy. More with whole virus vaccine. Therefore, not indicated in children.
- **Live attenuated vaccine**
  - Can be given in 2–49 yrs of age group. Trivalent, intranasal spray as single dose.
  - Not indicated in children less than two years of age, and in pregnant women.
- **Newer vaccine**
  - *Split virus:* Several injections are given
  - *Neuraminidase specific:* Subunit vaccine containing only N antigen
  - Recombinant vaccine

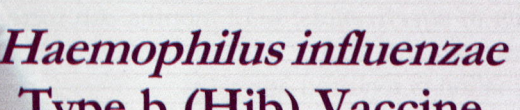

18

Haemophilus influenzae
Type b (Hib) Vaccine

- Capsulated *Haemophilus influenzae* has 6 serotypes of which type b is most important in causing serious disease. Most infections occur in children <2 years of age.
- Hib vaccine administration reduces Hib meningitis by 90% and Hib pneumonia by 1/3rd in children.
- Every year, in the world, about 3,70,000 children less than 5 years of age die due to Hib infection. Of these, 20% children are reported to be from India.
- Tamil Nadu was the 1st state to vaccinate all newborns by introducing pentavalent vaccines. Kerala also was included in this initiative.
- *Pentavalent vaccine prevents against 5 diseases:* Diphtheria, pertussis, tetanus, Hib and hepatitis B.
- *Type of vaccine:* Conjugated freeze-dried vaccine.
- The Hib capsular polysaccharide (polyribosylribitol phosphate or PRP) is conjugated with one of the following carriers:
- CRM_{197} mutant *Corynebacterium diphtheriae* toxin protein: HbOC
- Outer membrane protein complex of *N. meningitidis* strain B_{11}: PRP-OMP
- *Tetanus toxoid:* PRP-T
- Only HbOc and PRP-T are available in India.
- *Route and site:* Intramuscular injection. Anterolateral aspect of the thigh in infants, or into the deltoid muscles of older children
- *Dose:* 0.5 ml
- *Schedule*
  - *Newborns:* 4 doses—6,10, 14 wks, booster—12–18 months
  - *6–12 months:* 2 primary doses four weeks apart and 1 booster
  - *12–15 months:* 1 primary dose and 1 booster

- > *15 months–5 years:* Single dose
- *>5 years:* Not recommended

Booster should be given after a gap of at least 2 months.

- **Indications:** All children (6 weeks to 5 years) are immunized under NIS by pentavalent vaccine in selected states.
- All individuals with functional or anatomic hyposplenia irrespective of age should be given Hib vaccine.
- **Storage temperature:** The freeze-dried vaccine should be stored between +2°C and +8°C, protected from light.
- **Contraindications:** Known hypersensitivity to any component of the vaccine or a severe reaction to a previous dose. Children infected with Human Immunodeficiency Virus (HIV) both asymptomatic and symptomatic, should be immunized with Hib vaccine according to standard schedules.
- **Vaccine interactions:** Individuals receiving immunosuppressive therapy (e.g. corticotropin, corticosteroids) may have a diminished antibody response to immunization with Haemophilus type b conjugate vaccine.
- Hib vaccine can be given safely and effectively at the same time as BCG, DTP, measles, polio vaccines (OPV or IPV), HBV or yellow fever vaccines. It can be administered simultaneously with a different inactivated or live vaccine but separately at different sites.
- **Adverse effects:** Pain and tenderness at the injection site may occur within 24 hours of vaccination.

FAQs

Q. Is *H. influenzae* offered under UIP in India?

Ans. Yes, recently *H. influenzae* has been included under UIP in India. It is available as a pentavalent vaccine in combination with diphtheria, pertussis, tetanus and hepatitis B.

Q. Can we use *H. influenzae* vaccine from different manufacturers to complete the series of vaccination?

Ans. Yes, Hib conjugate vaccines licensed for use in infants are interchangeable. The series may be completed with any vaccine licensed for infants.

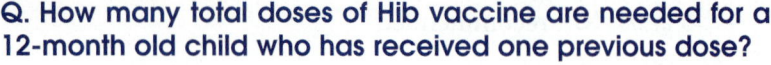

Q. How many total doses of Hib vaccine are needed for a 12-month old child who has received one previous dose?

Ans. A 12-month old child who has received only one previous dose prior to the first birthday would now need one dose of any conjugate Hib vaccine, and a second dose 2 months later.

Pneumococcal Vaccine

- **Type of vaccine:** Two types of vaccine are available: **Polysaccharide vaccines** which provides short duration of protection and **Polysaccharide-protein conjugate vaccines** with better herd immunity and increased immunogenicity in children <2 yrs.

Differences between the two vaccines are listed in Table 19.1:

Table 19.1: Differences between polysaccharide and polysaccharide conjugate pneumococcal vaccine		
Characteristics	Polysaccharide vaccine	Polysaccharide conjugate vaccine
Type	Polyvalent polysaccharide	Polyvalent polysaccharide conjugate vaccine
Strain	23 serotypes contained in the vaccine (1, 2, 3, 4, 5, 6B, 7F, 8, 9N, 9V, 10A, 11A, 12F, 14, 15B, 17F, 18C, 19F, 19A, 20, 22F, 23F, and 33F)	13 serotypes contained in the vaccine (1, 3, 4, 5, 6A, 6B, 7F, 9V, 14, 18C, 19A, 19F, 23F)
Conjugate	None	Conjugated to non-toxic diphtheria cross-reactive material (CRM 197) also contains adjuvant but no thiomersal
Storage	2–8°C	2–8°C; must not be frozen
Age of administration	>2 yrs and adults	<2 yrs who are at increased risk for pneumococcal disease or among persons ≥50 years of age
Route	Intramuscular or sub-cutaneous injection	Intramuscular or subcu-taneous

Contd...

Table 19.1: Differences between polysaccharide and polysaccharide conjugate pneumococcal vaccine (*Contd...*)

Characteristics	Polysaccharide vaccine	Polysaccharide conjugate vaccine
Site	Deltoid muscle	Anterolateral aspect of thigh in infants or deltoid muscle in children
Dose	0.5 ml	0.5 ml
Schedule	Single dose	6, 10, 14 wks and booster at 12–15 months
Revaccination	Routine revaccination is not recommended	
Development of immunity	After 7 days of the last dose	
Efficacy of vaccine	50–85% effective on preventing invasive pneumococcal disease	75% effective
Herd immunity	No	Yes
Adverse reaction	Pain/tenderness, swelling/ induration at the site of injection, fatigue (13.2%), and myalgia	Reduced appetite, irritability, fever
Precautions	Person with thrombocytopenia or any coagulation disorder, HIV infection, malignancy, pregnancy and lactation	
C/I	Allergic reaction	Previous history of hypersensitivity

FAQs

Q. If an unvaccinated child ≥7 months comes to your clinic for pneumococcal vaccination, how many doses should be given?

Ans. Pneumococcal vaccination schedule for previously unvaccinated children ≥7 months of age

Age at first dose	Total number of 0.5 ml dose
7–11 months of age	3 doses: 2 doses at least 4 weeks apart; third dose after 1 yr birthday, separated from the second dose by at least 2 months.

Age at first dose	Total number of 0.5 ml dose
12–23 months of age	2 doses at least 2 months apart
≥ 24 months–5 years of age (prior to 6th birthday)	1 dose

Minimum age for administering first dose is ideally 2 months but can be given at 6 weeks of age. Minimum interval between two doses for children vaccinated at age <12 months is 4 weeks, whereas it is 2 months (8 weeks) for those vaccinated at age >12 months.

Q What are the indications of pneumococcal polysaccharide vaccine (PPSV23)?

Ans. Pneumococcal polysaccharide vaccine is recommended for:
- Age 65 years and older
- Chronic pulmonary disease

Q. If a patient has had laboratory-confirmed pneumococcal pneumonia, does he or she still need to be vaccinated with PCV13 and/ or PPSV23?

Ans. Yes, as is true for other polyvalent vaccines such as OPV, etc. a disease state does not provide immunity against all the serotypes of the bacteria/virus. Similarly, infection with pneumococcus will not guarantee immunity against all the 90 known serotypes of pneumococcus. Vaccination will ensure protection against at least 23 serotypes (PPSV23) or 13 serotypes (PCV13). Therefore, patients who require vaccination should be vaccinated irrespective of their previous disease status.

Q. What are the recommendations regarding routine use of PCV10/13 in healthy children more than 5 years of age?

Ans. Routine use of PCV10/13 is not recommended for healthy children aged more than 5 years.

20

Rotavirus Vaccine

- Rotavirus accounts for 31–87% of health care associated gastroenteritis out of which one-third is severe.
- *In 1999:* RotaShield was withdrawn from the market because of its association with intussusceptions.
- Later 2 live attenuated oral vaccines were introduced in 2006.
- **Monovalent human rotavirus vaccine (RV1/Rotarix):**
  - *Type of vaccine:* Live attenuated human strain 89–12 [type G1P1 (8)] rotavirus. Available as lyophilized powder which is to be reconstituted with a diluent.
  - No preservatives.
  - *Storage temperature:* 2–8°C
  - *Route and schedule:* Orally 2 doses (1 ml each), 4 weeks apart. Start at 6–12 wks and complete by 16–24 wks.
- *Pentavalent bovine human reassortant vaccine (RV5/Rota Teq):*
  - *Type of vaccine:* Reassortant vaccine, liquid form, no reconstitution is required
  - No preservative or thiomersal.
  - *Storage temperature:* 2–8°C
  - *Route and schedule:* Orally 3 doses: 2, 4 and 6 months. Start at 6–12 wks; *not later:* Complete before 32 wks.
- *Absolute contraindications*
  - Severe allergic reaction to a previous dose.
  - History of intussusceptions.

FAQs

Q. Can rotavirus vaccine be offered during breastfeeding?

Ans. Yes. It can be offered as per schedule when child is on breastfeeding. However, as is with OPV, hot fluids should be refrained for at least half an hour following the administration of the vaccine.

Q. What should be done if the infant regurgitates or spits out the vaccine?

Ans. Repeat administration is not required generally, but it may be indicated by some manufacturers.

Remaining doses should be administered as per the schedule.

Q. Is it safe to give rotavirus vaccines of different types in the immunization schedule?

Ans. Ideally the schedule of rotavirus vaccination should be completed with same type of vaccine. However, in case of non-availability or non-remembrance of the vaccine type given earlier, another type may be given to complete the vaccination.

21

Typhoid Vaccine

Active Immunization

- Does not give 100% protection
- Lowers the incidence and seriousness of the infection
- Recommended for:
  - >2 yrs of age
  - Endemic area residents
  - Household contacts
  - At risk groups: School children, hospital staff
  - Travelers to endemic areas, *melas* and *yatras*
- *Types of vaccine:* Two types of vaccines are available.
  Differences between the characteristic of both vaccines is given in Table 21.1:

Table 21.1: Differences between Ty21a vaccine and Vi polysaccharide vaccine for typhoid vaccination

Characteristics	Ty21a vaccine	Vi polysaccharide vaccine
Type	Live	Killed; subunit vaccine
Strain	Ty2 *S. typhi* mutated genes	Ty2 *S. typhi*
Forms	Capsule form (for >5 years old) and liquid suspension	Injections (25 µg of purified polysaccharide in 0.5 ml of vaccine)
Storage temperature	2–8°C; stable for 14 days at 25°C	2–8°C; stable for 6 months at 37°C and 2 yrs at 22°C
Age of administration	> 2 yrs	> 2 yrs
Route	Oral	S/C or IM
Dose	3 doses regime on 1, 3 and 5th day; in some countries	Single dose

Contd...

Table 21.1: Differences between Ty21a vaccine and Vi polysaccharide vaccine for typhoid vaccination (*Contd...*)

Characteristics	Ty21a vaccine	Vi polysaccharide vaccine
	it is given as 4 doses regimen on 1, 3, 5, 7th day	
Revaccination	1 yr (travelers); 3 yrs (endemic)	Every 3 yr
Development of immunity	After 7 days of last dose	After 7 days
Precautions	Proguanil and antibiotics s/b stopped 3 days before to 3 days after the vaccine. Can be given to HIV +ve individuals with CD4 count >200/mm^3	None
C/I	Immunodeficiency, acute febrile illness, and acute intestinal infection	Previous history of hypersensitivity

A Vi polysaccharide conjugate vaccine is in the phase of development and trial for use in younger children below one year of age.

FAQs

Q. What is 'TAB' vaccine and why was TAB vaccine discontinued?

Ans. "TAB" vaccine stand for vaccine combining typhoid and paratyphoid A and B antigens. TAB vaccine was discontinued because of the following reasons:

a. It was observed that combining paratyphoid A and B antigens with typhoid vaccine increases the risk of vaccine reactions, while the side effects of monovalent vaccines are less.

b. Lack of known efficacy for the paratyphoid A component of TAB vaccine

c. Typhoid infection from paratyphoid B component is epidemiologically less relevant in our country.

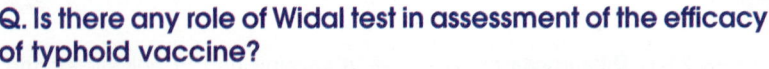

Q. Is there any role of Widal test in assessment of the efficacy of typhoid vaccine?

Ans. No, there is no role of Widal test in assessment of the efficacy of typhoid vaccine since anti-H and anti-O have poor correlation with efficacy and potency of the typhoid vaccine. However, efficacy of typhoid vaccine can be judged by the Vi antibody level.

Q. Can we administer the typhoid vaccine to those who have already suffered from typhoid fever?

Ans. The development of immunity after natural infection of typhoid is being reported but not with all the cases of typhoid and this could also be predicted by relapses and recurrences of typhoid fever after the episode of disease. Therefore, we can administer the vaccine, even after typhoid fever. However, there is no clear recommendation on when to vaccinate. The vaccine can be administered after 2–3 months of recovery as the antibodies may interfere with the vaccine, if the vaccine is administered earlier.

Q. Is it worthwhile to advise the typhoid vaccine among household contacts?

Ans. Yes, vaccination among household contacts can be advised as the disease may spread among other household members, although the spread of disease through this method is not a common mode of transmission.

Q. Can the vaccine be safely given in severely malnourished children?

Ans. Yes, both killed and live attenuated vaccine can be offered to malnourished children, however, response from the vaccine reported may be poor.

Q. Can the vaccine be safely given in pregnancy?

Ans. It is better to avoid the typhoid vaccine during pregnancy, however, if the lady is travelling in a country where typhoid disease is a problem, then the killed variety of typhoid vaccine can be administered to her. Live attenuated typhoid vaccine should not be administered among pregnant women.

Q. What will happen if oral typhoid vaccine is administered in patients receiving antibiotics?

Ans. The vaccine should not be administered to individuals receiving sulfonamides and antibiotics since these agents may be active against the vaccine strain and prevent a sufficient of multiplication to occur thus hampering a protective immune response.

Q. What precaution is needed for the person while receiving oral typhoid vaccine?

Ans. The oral typhoid vaccine is given in the form of a capsule which is to be swallowed approximately 1 hour before a meal with cold or lukewarm (temperature not to exceed body temperature, e.g. 37°C).

Q. A person has planned to travel in an area which is endemic for typhoid. As an consultant for his vaccination against typhoid, how long before his travel to area will you advise the oral typhoid vaccine?

Ans. Immunization with typhoid vaccine should be completed at least 1 week prior to potential exposure to *S. typhi*, which means that last capsule should be swallowed 7 days prior to visit the area.

Q. For how long is the oral typhoid vaccine effective and how frequently should the boosters be given?

Ans. The optimum booster schedule for oral typhoid vaccine has not been determined. Efficacy has been shown to persist for 3–5 years.

22

Cholera Vaccine

Types of Vaccine

Parental (discontinued now) and oral vaccine.

A. *Parenteral Killed Vaccine*

- *Content:* 12000 vibrios of classical Ogawa and Inaba serotypes/ml
- *Discontinued.*
- *Protective value:* 50% for a period of 3–6 months. Does not prevent the development of carrier state.

Two new oral cholera vaccines which provide good protection for up to 3 years are now available for use by travelers.

B. *Oral Vaccine*

Cholera vaccine is not routinely recommended for healthy people. It is administered to residents of highly endemic areas and travellers to area of high-risk such as *melas*, disaster, etc.

1. WC/rBS (Dukoral)

- Killed whole-cell *V. cholerae* in combination with recombinant B subunit of cholera toxin.
- Given with a bicarbonate buffer
- *Storage:* Vaccine is stored at 2°C–8°C. It should not be freeze.
- *Schedule:* Given orally in 2 doses schedule, ≥7 days but <6 wks apart in those ≥6 yrs of age.

In 2–5 yrs: 3 doses. It should not be offered in <2 yrs of age and booster should be given every 2 yrs.

Provides cross immunity to enterotoxigenic *E. coli*, because of its similarity cholera toxin B.

- *Precautions:* Avoid food, drink and medicine 1 hour before and after the vaccination.

- Take the 2nd dose at least 1 week after the 1st dose and at least 1 week before starting your trip.

Possible side effects: Severe diarrhea with loss of water from the body, pain, stomach cramps, gurgling stomach, bloated stomach, stomach gas, allergic reactions and rarely reduced sense of taste

2. Sanchol and mORCVAX

- *Type:* Unlike dukoral, it does not contain B subunit toxin and therefore does not provide cross immunity to enterotoxigenic *E. coli.*
- Based on serogroup O1 and O139.
- *Schedule:* Orally, 2 doses, 14 days apart in ≥1 yr age
- *Storage:* Vaccine is stored at 2°C – 8°C. It should not be freeze.
- Since the efficacy and safety has not been evaluated among pregnant women and infants therefore not recommended for use in this group.
- *Mechanism of action:* When vaccine is administered orally, it induces an IgA antibody response similar to natural disease. These antibacterial antibodies prevent the bacteria from attaching to the intestinal wall thereby impeding the colonization of the *V. cholerae* O1 and O139 strains.
- *Adverse reaction:* Acute gastroenteritis, diarrhea, fever, vomiting, rash, cough, dryness of mouth, etc.

CVD 103-HgR vaccine (no longer produced)

- Live attenuated, genetically manipulated classical *V. cholerae* strain.
- Single dose.
- 80% protection against El Tor.
- Ab and proguanil s/b avoided 1 wk before to 1 wk after the vaccine.
- Start of protection ≥8 days, booster at 6 months.

FAQs

Q. Why was parenteral killed vaccine of typhoid discontinued?

Ans. The reasons for discontinuation of vaccines were:

- The protective value of vaccine was 50% for a period of 3–6 months.
- Does not prevent the development of carrier state.

Q. Is it necessary to have the cholera vaccination certificate for international travel?

Ans. No country requires proof of cholera vaccination as a condition for entry, therefore international certificate of cholera vaccination is no longer required.

Q. A person is visiting an area which is cholera affected, he has already received the required cholera vaccine doses. What other precautions will you advise to the person?

Ans. As the cholera vaccines does not provide 100% protection, therefore adherence to dietary measures and basic hygienic precautions will be advised to the person besides the vaccination.

Q. Is it useful to offer cholera vaccine at the time of epidemics?

Ans. No, it is not useful to offer the cholera vaccine during epidemics as it gives only false sense of protection from cholera. The prevention of cholera during the epidemics is ensured by high standards of sanitation and hygiene and by giving safe water for drinking purpose.

Q. Why is cholera vaccine used along with bicarbonate buffer?

Ans. Cholera vaccine is used along with the buffer solution, as it protects the vaccine from the gastric acid of stomach.

Q. Can we offer Shanchol vaccine to a person suffering from cholera?

Ans. No, this vaccine is not a substitute for therapy in case an individual is suspected to be suffering from cholera or showing signs and symptoms of acute episode of gastrointestinal disease. It is only used for prevention purpose.

Q. Can we offer the vaccine parenterally?

Ans. No, vaccine should be offered orally only and should not be offered parenterally.

23

Rabies Vaccine

Rabies is one of the few diseases where the vaccine works even after the exposure (other diseases are tetanus, hepatitis B, measles).

Types of Rabies Vaccine

1. Nervous Tissue Vaccine

a. Nervous tissue vaccine (NTV) also known as semple vaccine or beta propionolactone (BPL) vaccine is an inactivated vaccine produced in sheep or goat brain tissue (therefore known as nervous tissue vaccine)—usually 5% emulsion is reported to be having neuroparalytic effects—1 : 200 to 1 : 1600 and lethality up to 14%.

Characteristics are:

- Given deep subcutaneously daily for 7–10 days
- Dose will depend upon category of wound and company who has developed the vaccine
- Site is anterior abdominal wall

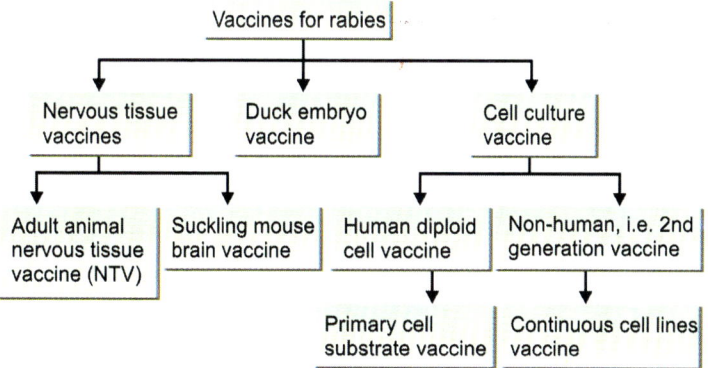

b. Suckling mouse brain (Fuenzalida) →devoid of neuroparalytic effects due to its low myelin sheath content.

Now the vaccines are no longer used in India

2. *Duck Embryo Vaccine*

3. *Cell Culture Vaccine*

The major disadvantage of the cell culture vaccine is their cost

a. Human origin is human diploid cell vaccine (1967)—based on the Pitman-Moore L503 strain.

b. 2nd generation vaccine from non-human sources is chick fibroblast or vero cell line vaccine.

- Purified chick cell embryo vaccine (Rabipur)—uses Flury LEP-25 strain
- Non-tumorigenic continuous/vero cells cell lines vaccine (Indirab)—uses Wistar strain.

Prophylaxis against rabies: There are three types of prophylaxis available for the prevention of rabies.

i. *Post-exposure prophylaxis:* Best achieved by combined administration of a single dose of rabies immunoglobulin

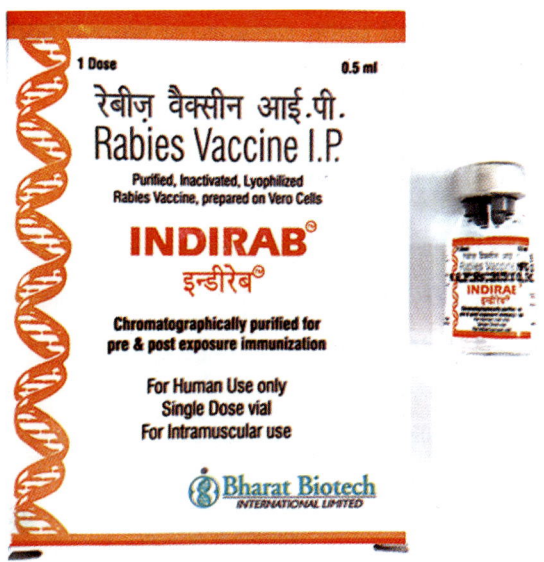

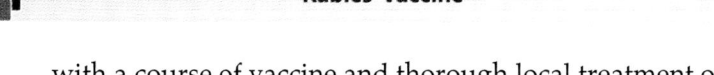

with a course of vaccine and thorough local treatment of the wound depending upon the class of bite.

ii. Pre-exposure prophylaxis

iii. Post-exposure prophylaxis in those who have already received the rabies vaccine in the past: No Ig required.

Steps for prevention of rabies in **post-exposure prophylaxis,** i.e. after the bite by an animal.

- Thorough washing with soap and running water for at least 15 minutes should be done. In case of puncture wounds, catheters may be used for washing the deeper areas.

- No stitches should be made initially as it may cause additional trauma and promote the penetration of rabies virus in deeper tissues thereby shortening the incubation period.

- Thorough debridement of the wound is to be done. If the stitches are essential, they should be applied after 24–48 hrs under cover of immunoglobulin (delayed primary suturing).

- Chemical treatment by virucidal agents like 70% alcohol, 0.01% aqueous iodine or providone iodine.

- Tetanus toxoid and antibiotics as required might be given.

- *Passive immunization*
  - Rabies immunoglobulin (RIG) to be injected thoroughly into and around the wound. The two types of immunoglobulin that are available for use are:
    - *Human rabies immunoglobulin:* 20 U/kg body weight, up to a maximum dose of 1500 IU. or
    - *Horse antirabies serum:* 40 u/kg body weight, up to a maximum dose of 3000 IU.
  - The remaining immunoglobulin should be injected IM at a site away from the vaccine site.
  - RIG may be diluted with normal saline if the amount for infiltration of all wounds is insufficient.
  - RIG can be administered up to maximum of 7 days of start of vaccination against rabies.
  - It is *not* indicated in people who have been vaccinated earlier for rabies (Tables 23.1 and 23.2).

Table 23.1: Exposure category and details

Category	Type of contact	Recommended PEP
Class I	• Touching or feeding of animal • Licks on intact skin	None, if reliable case history about the vaccination status of animal is available
Class II	• Nibbling of uncovered skin • Minor scratches or abrasions without oozing of blood	Wound management, administer vaccine
Class III	• Single or multiple bites or scratches licks on broken skin • Contamination of mucous membrane with saliva, exposure to bats	Wound management, rabies immunoglobulin and vaccine

Table 23.2: Rabies active vaccination schedule

Type of prophylaxis	Schedule
PEP (Essen schedule)	Day 0, 3, 7, 14, 28 (IM)
• Abbreviated multisite schedule	Day 0 (2 sites), 7, 21
• 2 site ID schedule (2-2-2-0-2-0) (AKA updated Thai Red Cross Regimen)	Day 0, 3, 7, 28 (at 2 sites each)
Pre-exposure prophylaxis	Day 0, 7, 28 (IM/ID)
Post-exposure prophylaxis of previously vaccinated*	
• Unknown antibody titer	Day 0, 3, 7
• Antibody titer >0.5 IU/ml	Day 0, 3

*Day 0 is the day of commencement of vaccination

- *Dose*
  - Human diploid cell vaccine, purified chick embryo cell vaccine, purified duck embryo vaccine: 1.0 ml
  - Purified vero cell vaccine: 0.5 ml
- *Route of vaccination:* Usually IM in anterolateral aspect of mid-thigh in children and deltoid in adults. It should not be offered in gluteal region since the absorption might be inhibited.
- It is offered by the government free of cost in health institutions with a minimum of 50 patients of animal bite per day.

Protection of Dogs

- Rabies among dogs can be mainly prevented by giving the chick embryo vaccine.
- The schedule usually offered is on 0th day, 1 month later and booster at 1 year.

Oral Rabies Vaccine

- Oral rabies vaccine (Raboral) is available for use among wild animals like raccoons, foxes, dogs, etc.

Other Important Points to Remember

- Recently introduction of oral vaccines for the immunization of foxes is a great advancement in rabies prophylaxis of wildlife.
- Rabies in dogs is of 2 types:
  - Furious (mad dog syndrome)
  - Dumb rabies
- Rabies among dogs can be mainly prevented by giving the chick embryo vaccine.
- *Control of urban rabies:* By elimination of stray dogs and swift mass immunization of at least 80% of dogs (preferred method).

FAQs ON DOG BITE

Q. Why do we have to observe a dog/cat for 10 days after the bite?

Ans. Since the period of communicability of rabies among dog varies from 3 to 5 days before onset of disease and last for about 5–6 days, therefore the observation of dog is usually done for 10 days. If the dog remains healthy and does not develop symptoms of rabies during the 10 days of observation period, post-exposure prophylaxis is not required.

Q. Is it necessary to observe the other animals also for 10 days?

Ans. The observation period of 10 days is valid for dogs and cats only, since the natural history of rabies in other animals is not fully understood.

Q. What should be done if dog/cat remains healthy after 10 days?

Ans. We can modify the treatment by converting the post-exposure prophylaxis to pre-exposure prophylaxis, i.e. we can skip the 14th day dose and offer on 28th day if we are following the IM schedule but no modification should be done if we are offering the vaccine through ID route.

Q. If a person is bitten by an untraceable stray dog, what should be done?

Ans. All the wounds by untraceable animals are considered as Class III wounds and should be considered for full PEP.

Q. Is there any difference in management between animal bite by a provoked or unprovoked dog?

Ans. No. Provoked bite is defined as the bite by a dog when he/she is excited by activity like pulling the meal from the dog once being offered, or putting the feet over the tail of a dog, etc. PEP should be administered irrespective of the provocation status. There is no difference between provoked bite and unprovoked bite by an animal, both types of bites should be followed by a full PEP.

Q. Bites made by which animals should not be considered for rabies vaccination?

Ans. The bite by the domestic rodents, squirrel, hare and rabbits does not require PEP. The management in such situation requires only washing of wound with application of antiseptics and topical antibiotics.

Q. Is there any possibility of transmitting rabies by a pet vaccinated dog?

Ans. Yes, the efficacy of rabies vaccine among dogs is not 100%.

WOUND

Q. What should be done if rabies wound requires stitching?

Ans. Stitching in rabies wound should be avoided for at least 24–48 hours. This is because if we stitch the wound earlier it causes additional trauma favoring deeper penetration of the virus and quicker adherence to the nerve endings. Minimal number of stitches should be applied after 24–48 hours and under the cover of local immunoglobulin.

RABIES VACCINATION

Q. A person is bitten by a dog. He had received the pre-exposure prophylaxis earlier, what is next line of management?

Ans. A person who has received the pre-exposure/post-exposure prophylaxis within past 2 years, can be offered a schedule of 0, 3, 7. However, if more than 2 years have been elapsed since the person has either received pre- or post-exposure prophylaxis then full PEP should be offered to person.

Q. A child has recovered from chickenpox/measles. Can we give rabies vaccine to him/her?

Ans. Rabies is 100% fatal and hence there is no contraindication to PEP at all.

Q. Can a rabies vaccine be offered to pregnant/lactating mother?

Ans. All rabies vaccines are known to be safe during pregnancy. Besides pregnant women with history of animal bite are susceptible to rabies and should be given PEP.

Q. Why rabies vaccine is not offered in gluteal region?

Ans. Gluteal region is rich in fat which absorbs the vaccine and hence it suppresses the immune response. In children, it should be given in anterolateral aspect of thigh while in adults it is administered at deltoid.

Q. Why rabies vaccine should be started as soon as possible?

Ans. The basis to start the vaccine at earliest is to immunize or protect the individual before the rabies virus reaches the nervous system.

Q. Is there any drug which can interfere with the production of rabies antibody?

Ans. Choloroquine has been found to interfere with the production of the rabies antibody, therefore it should be avoided.

Q. Which rabies vaccines are currently use in India?

Ans. At present in our country we are mainly using cell culture vaccine (CCV) or purified duck embryo vaccine (PDEV).

Q. Can we change the brand of vaccine during the course of rabies vaccination?

Ans. No, ideally it should not be changed.

Q. Can we switch over from one route to another route during the rabies vaccination course?

Ans. No, there are no scientifically proven records on vaccine immunogenicity once the schedule has been changed.

RABIES IMMUNOGLOBULIN

Q. How much time gap can be allowed between bite by an animal and serotherapy?

Ans. Ideally a person should be offered the immunoglobulin immediately after the bite however it can be offered up to 7 days (or even thereafter also) after the bite by an animal. However, it should be given within an interval of 24 hours of the first dose of the vaccine.

Q. What is the basis of offering the RIG around the wound?

Ans. The RIG is given around the wound because of the property of RIG to bind with virus which results in loss of infectivity of virus.

Q. What is the dose of RIG?

Ans. The dose of RIG should be 20 IU/kg of body weight in case human RIG and 40 IU/kg in case of equine RIG.

Q. What precautions should be taken while offering the RIG?

Ans. RIG should be brought to room temperature (25°C to 30°C) before administration to the patient.

Multiple needle injections into the wound/s should be avoided.

After all the wound/s has/have been infiltrated, if any volume of RIG is remaining, it should be administered by deep intramuscular injection at a site distant from the vaccine injection site.

In those circumstances where multiple site injury is present and enough volume of the vaccine is not available, it is advisable to dilute the calculated volume of RIG in sterile normal saline to a volume sufficient to infiltrate all the wounds.

The total recommended dose of RIG must not be exceeded as it may suppress the antibody production stimulated by the anti-rabies vaccine.

Q. Can we administer RIG for multiple times?

Ans. Rabies immunoglobulin for passive immunization is administered only once, preferably within 24 hours after the exposure, i.e. on day 0 along with the first dose of anti-rabies vaccine.

Q. A dog bite case has presented after 6 days of bite. Is it worth to administer the RIG?

Ans. If RIG was not administered when ARV was begun, it can be administered up to the seventh day after the administration of the first dose of ARV. Beyond the seventh day, it is not indicated as it may interfere with the production of antibodies.

24

Japanese Encephalitis Vaccine

Type of vaccines: Five types of vaccines are available for vaccination against JE.

1. **Vero cell culture derived SA 14-14-2 inactivated vaccine.**
   - **Minimum age of vaccination**: 1 year
   - **Dose, route and schedule**
     - For children between 1 and 3 years of age: 0.25 ml, 2 doses, IM on day 0 and 28.
     - For adults: 0.5 ml.

2. **Vero cell culture derived, 821564XY, inactivated vaccine**
   - *Minimum age of vaccination:* 1 year
   - *Dose, route and schedule:* 0.5 ml, 2 doses, IM at 4 weeks interval.

3. **Live attenuated cell culture derived vaccine SA 14-14-2**
   - *Dose:* 0.5 ml, 2 doses
   - *Route:* Subcutaneous
   - *Age:* 8 months and 2 years. Booster at 7 years.
   - *Storage temperature:* Heat stable. Can be stored at 37°C for 7–10 days.
   - **Adverse effects:** Fever, local reactions, rash, and irritability.

4. **Live attenuated recombinant vaccine SA 14-14-2**
   Single dose followed by a single booster at an interval of 1 year.

5. **Mouse brain derived (Nakyama or Beijing starin)**
   - *Dose:* 2 doses (4 weeks apart), 0.5 ml among children <3 yrs while 1 ml to those above 3 years, booster after 1 year and subsequently every 3-year interval until the age of 10–15 years
   - *Route:* Subcutaneously
   - Best used in inter-epidemic period
   - *Immunity:* 1 month after 2nd dose

JE vaccine should not be used as an "outbreak response vaccine"

FAQs

Q. What are the adverse effects following JE vaccination?

Ans. JE vaccination may cause local reactions such as pain, swelling, redness at injection site and low grade fever, myalgia and GI upset in about 20% of the vaccines. The rare vaccine reactions include neurologic events such as encephalitis, encephalopathy and peripheral neuropathy at a frequency of $1–2.3/10^6$ vaccines. The treatment consists of symptomatic and supportive care.

Q. How many days earlier should a traveler to an endemic area be vaccinated with JE vaccine?

Ans. A traveler should receive the last dose of JE vaccine at least 10 days before commencement of travel to an endemic area for ensuring an adequate immune response.

Q. What is the effectiveness of the vaccine?

Ans. Complete vaccination has 90% effectiveness. However, other protective measures such as personal protection with clothing, mosquito repellants, bed nets, etc. should be practiced scrupulously.

Q. How long does the protection last after vaccination?

Ans. The protection lasts for at least 2 years after which boosters are required.

Q. Is JE vaccine administered under routine immunization in National Immunization Schedule in India?

Ans. JE has been included under NIS as a routine immunization vaccine in selected endemic districts at the age of 16–24 months after the catchup campaign in which it is given to all susceptible individuals.

25

Vaccines for Yellow Fever, Leptospirosis, Kyasanur Forest Disease, and Brucellosis

YELLOW FEVER

- *Type of vaccine and strain:* 17D strain vaccine, live attenuated freeze-dried
- *Dose, route and site:* 0.5 ml/SC or IM at lateral aspect of upper arm or anterolateral aspect of mid-thigh in young children
- *Storage temperature:* Should be stored at 2–8°C and should *not* be frozen.
- It is heat labile after reconstitution and should be used within one hour of reconstitution.
- Cholera vaccine should be given at least 3 wks apart as it interferes with antibody production.
- *Immunity:* Starts after 10 days, revaccinate after 10 years
- *Adverse effects*
  - *Mild:* Fever and myalgia
  - *Severe:* Immediate hypersensitivity reactions, neurologic disease, viscerotopic disease. Adverse effects are commoner in elderly and in infants <6 months of age.
- The vaccine is not indicated in India for routine vaccination; it is required for travelers to sub-Saharan Africa and South American countries.
- Minimum age of vaccination is 9 months.
- Can be used in pregnant women if benefit outweighs the risk.

LEPTOSPIROSIS

Immunization is done for pets as well as persons who are at high risk for contracting leptospirosis.

KYASANUR FOREST DISEASE

Vaccine—killed KFD vaccine.

BRUCELLOSIS (AKA UNDULENT FEVER, MALTA FEVER OR MEDITERRANEAN FEVER)

Vaccine is available only for *B. abortus*.

26

Plague Vaccine

- *Type of vaccine:* Formalin killed
- *Route:* SC or IM
- *Immunity:* For 6 months
- *Indications*
  1. All laboratory and field personnel working with Y. *pestis* or plague-infected rodents in lab or engaged in aerosol experiments with Y. *pestis*.
  2. Persons engaged in field operations in areas with enzootic plague where preventing exposure is not possible (such as some disaster areas).
- *Primary vaccination schedule*
  - Adults and children ≥11 years: 3 doses of vaccine.
    - The first dose, 1.0 ml, is followed by the second dose, 0.2 ml, 4 weeks later. The third dose, 0.2 ml, is administered 6 months after the first dose.
    - In case of an accelerated schedule: 3 doses of 0.5 ml each, administered at least 1 week apart, may be given. The efficacy of this schedule has not been determined.
  - Children <10 years old: 3 doses, but the doses are smaller.
- *Booster doses*
  - 3 booster doses should be given at approximately 6-month intervals, if there is continued exposure. Thereafter, booster doses at 1–2-year intervals, can be offered depending on the degree of continuing exposure.
- *Adverse effects*
  - *Mild reactions:* General malaise, headache, fever, mild lymphadenopathy, and erythema and induration at the injection site in about 10% of recipients.
  - *Rare reactions:* Sensitivity reactions and sterile abscess.

- **Precautions and contraindications**
  - Known hypersensitivity to any of the components, such as beef protein, soya, casein, and phenol.
  - Severe local or systemic reactions to previous plague vaccine
  - Should not be used during pregnancy unless there is a substantial risk of infection.

27

Human Papillomavirus (HPV) Vaccine

Table 27.1: Differences between bivalent and quadrivalent human papillomavirus viccines

Type of vaccine (VL particles)	Bivalent	Quadrivalent
Type of vaccine	Recombinant DNA vaccines, contain HPV L1 protein	
Protection against serotypes	HPV 16, 18 related infections	HPV 16, 18, 6, 11 related infections
Adjuvant	ASO_4	Aluminum hydroxide
Dose	0.5 ml	
Number of doses	3	
Injection site	Deltoid	
Route	Intramuscular	
Age and schedule	0, 1, 6 months	0, 2, 6 months
	Minimum age for giving first dose of vaccine: 10–12 yrs. Minimum dosage interval between doses 1 and 2 is 4 weeks and between 2 and 3rd dose is 12 weeks	
Booster	Not recommended at present	
Vaccine efficacy	95% protection against types 16, 18 related *Cervical Intraepithelial Neoplasia* 2/3 and *Adenocarcinoma in situ*	
Contraindications	History of 'immediate' hypersensitivity or severe allergic reaction to yeast or to any vaccine component. Should be postponed in women with an acute febrile illness/pregnancy	
Adverse reactions	Local pain, swelling, erythema and fever after vaccination. Syncope is common. Therefore, vaccine is to be administered in sitting/lying down position and the vaccine should be observed for 15 mins after vaccination.	
Storage	Store between +2°C and +8°C (vaccine must not be frozen)	

- Vaccination "before" adolescence is better than "after" adolescence in prevention of carcinoma cervix.
- Carcinoma cervix should be prevented by a combination of screening and vaccination strategies. Screening for pre-cancerous stages and appropriate treatment is very effective.
- Vaccines are protective against specific serotypes of viruses only and do not provide significant cross immunity to other serotypes. Also they are not useful once the neoplastic process has been initiated.

FAQs

Q. What are the common adverse effects of HPV vaccines?

Ans. Common adverse effects of HPV vaccines include mild local reactions such as pain, redness and swelling at the site of injection. Some individuals also complain of fever, headache, nausea, myalgia or joint pain. Fainting attacks may also occur in some individuals. These attacks may be prevented by lying down for 15 minutes after the vaccination.

Q. What are the benefits of HPV vaccination?

Ans. HPV vaccination affords 95% protection against types 16, 18 related *Cervical Intraepithelial Neoplasia* 2/3 and *Adenocarcinoma in situ*.

Q. For how long HPV vaccine will provide protection?

Ans. HPV vaccine is found to provide protection for at least 8 years and some report that the protection is lifelong.

Q. Which will provide better immune response: Natural infection or vaccination?

Ans. It has been found that vaccination provides higher level of antibodies than those produced by natural infection.

Q. What is the best time to give HPV vaccine: Before the start of sexual activity or after it?

Ans. HPV vaccines are most effective when given before the start of sexual activity, i.e. before any exposure to HPV. Any type of sexual activity whether oral/anal/genital predisposes to HPV infection and warrant HPV vaccine administration.

Q. Is it still important to get a Pap test after HPV vaccination?

Ans. Yes it is important to get screened for HPV infection by Pap test even after HPV vaccination since HPV vaccine provides protection against the most common 2–3 or maximum four serotypes of HPV only; the rest of the serotypes (total more than 40 in number) can still cause cervical cancer.

Q. Can someone who is sexually active, still get vaccinated against HPV?

Ans. It is never too late to get vaccinated with HPV vaccine since there is a possibility that the individual may not have been exposed to HPV infection yet. Giving HPV vaccination will provide protection against subsequent HPV infection.

Q. Can HPV vaccine be given to pregnant women?

Ans. HPV vaccine is not recommended for use in pregnant women; however administration of HPV vaccine accidently/ unknowingly does not warrant termination of pregnancy since no harmful effects on the baby has been documented.

Q. Can HPV vaccine be given to boys also?

Ans. The quadrivalent HPV vaccine has been shown to be effective in protecting against anogenital infections and external genital lesions such as genital warts caused due to HPV vaccine types in males 16–26 years of age. Giving HPV vaccine to boys will also contribute to increased protection among females due to the "herd immunity".

Q. Does HPV vaccine cause infertility?

Ans. No, the news about HPV vaccine causing infertility is not true and also not biologically plausible. Rather, by preventing cancer cervix it will contribute to increased fertility.

S. No.	Name	Form of vaccine	Schedule/ age	Dose	Route	Storage	Contra-indications	Efficacy effects	Adverse	Remarks
1.	BCG	LA, FD	Birth-14 days or at 6 wks	0.05 ml –0.1 ml	ID	2–8°C	CMI deficiency	0–80% (40%)	Ulceration, abscess, LN enlargement	Papule (2–3 wks) 4–8 mm n 5 wks-healing in 6–12 wks
2.	DPT	D and T-toxoid, P—killed	6,10,14 wks; booster 1.5 yrs	0.5 ml	Deep IM	2–8°C	Severe allergic reaction to DPT, encephalopathy progressive neurological deficit	D—90%, P—80%, T—almost 100%	Encephalitis and Reye's syndrome	Invalid contraindications of DPT are temperature <40°C family history of seizures, stable neurological conditions
3.	DT (no longer produced now)	Toxoid	Above 5 yrs 2 doses to 1 month interval; 1 booster only if DPT is given	0.5 ml	Deep IM	2–8°C	There are no as such hard contraindication	-	Fever, local swelling and pain	Nowadays at 5 years we are using DPT only
4.	OPV (Sabin)	LA	0,6,10, 14 wks	2 drops	Oral	–20°C (2 yr),	Persistent vomiting,	70–80%	None	Immunocompromised

Contd...

S. No.	Name	Form of vaccine	Schedule/age	Dose	Route	Storage	Contra-indications	Efficacy effects	Adverse	Remarks
					4°C (1 yr), room (1 m)	diarrhea				states
5.	IPV (Salk)	Killed	4 doses 6, 14,22 weeks and at 3.5 years	0.5 ml	S/C or IM	2–8°C	There are no as such hard contraindica-tion	100% effective after 2nd dose	None	Can be offered among immunocom-promised, recently included in UIP
6.	Hepatitis B	Killed, two types plasma derived and recom-binant	Various schedules, e.g. at birth, 6, 10 and 14 weeks or birth, 1 and 6 months or 0,6 wks and 14 wks, etc. All schedules are equally protective	0.5 ml	IM	4–8°C	Allergy to vaccine contents	15 years or life-long	Fever and local reaction like pain and swelling, soreness at the site of vaccine	Interruption of schedule does not require restarting instead person can take the vaccine as soon as he remember the dose

Contd...

S. No.	Name	Form of vaccine	Schedule/ age	Dose	Route	Storage	Contra-indications	Efficacy effects	Adverse	Remarks
7.	Chicken-pox	LA (OKA strain	12–18 months	0.5 ml single dose; 2 doses in >12 yrs	S/C, upper arm	−50°C and −15°C	Pregnancy, immuno-compromised persons, allergic to neomycin	Lifelong	Local reaction, seizure	Salicylates s/b avoided for 6 wks after
8.	Measles	LA, FD, Edmonston Zagreb strain	>9 months	0.5 ml	Subcu-taneous/ IM	Can be frozen or stored at 2–8°C	Pregnancy, acute illness, deficient CMI, steroids and immuno-suppressant, high fever, allergy to contents. Early stage HIV infection: Not contra-indication	Lifelong	Toxic shock syndrome	No preserva-tives (thiomersal) in measles vaccine, at 37°C—utilize in 1 hr and at 2–8°C—utilize in 6 hrs
9.	Rubella	LA, RA-27/3	After one year of age	0.5 ml	Subcu-taneous	Can be frozen or stored at 2–8°C	Pregnancy, immuno-compromised persons	Lifelong	Local reaction, thrombo phlebitis	Seizure, temporary pain and stiffness in the joints, temporary low platelet count

Contd...

S. No.	Name	Form of vaccine	Schedule/ age	Dose	Route	Storage	Contra-indications	Efficacy effects	Adverse	Remarks
10.	Mumps	LA, Jeryl Lynn, Leningrad-3, L- Zagreb and Urabe strain and RIT 4385	After one year of age	0.5 ml	IM	Can be frozen or stored at 2–8°C	Pregnancy, immunocompromised persons	Lifelong	Fever, febrile seizures, aseptic meningitis	Recently included in UIP in form of MMR
11.	Influenza	Killed	>6 months	0.5 ml	S/C	Stored at 2–8°C	Severe allergic reaction to egg, ever had Guillain-Barré syndrome	One year	Soreness, redness, or swelling where the shot was given, hoarseness, sore or red eyes, cough, itchiness, fever, aches	None
		Live	In 2–49 yrs of age	-	Intranasal spray	Stored at 2–8°C	Hypersensitivity to the active substances, immunocompromised persons, person receiving salicylates therapy	-	Nasal congestion/ rhinorrhea	None

Contd...

S. No.	Name	Form of vaccine	Schedule/ age	Dose	Route	Storage	Contra-indications	Efficacy effects	Adverse	Remarks
12.	Meningo-coccal meningitis	Capsular polysac-charide	> 2 years	Single dose, 0.5 ml	Subcu-taneously/ IM	2–8°C	Hypersensitivity to the active sub-stances	Short duration	Pain and redness at injection site, transient fever.	None
		Protein poly-saccharide conjugate vaccine	< 2 yrs age	0.5 ml	IM	2–8°C	Hypersensitivity to the active substances	-	Pain and red-ness at injection site	Recommended for travelers, safe in pregnancy
13.	Hib	Conjugated freeze-dried vaccine	Up to 5 years of age	<1 yr–4 doses-6, 10, 14 wks; booster 12–18 months; >1 yr Single dose; >2 yrs—not recomm-ended	SC among infants and deltoid muscles lateron/IM	+2°C– +8°C	Hypersensitivity to the active substances	Not known exactly but likely last up to 1.5 to 3.5 years	Pain and tenderness at the injection	None
14.	Pneumo-coccal	PPV23 nonconju-gate: Capsular Ag of 23	>2 years and adults	Single dose, 0.5 ml	IM	2–8°C	Hypersensitivity to the active substances	After 7 days of the last dose	Pain/tender-ness, swelling/ induration at the site of injection	None

Contd...

S. No.	Name	Form of vaccine	Schedule/ age	Dose	Route	Storage	Contra-indications	Efficacy effects	Adverse	Remarks
		serotypes								
		Polyvalent polysaccharide conjugate vaccine Ag of 13 serotypes	Infants and >2 years of age	6, 10, 14 wks and booster at 12–15 months	IM	2–8°C	Hypersensitivity to the active substances	After 7 days of the last dose	Reduced appetite, irritability, fever	None
15.	Japanese encephalitis	Five types of vaccines are available	≥1 year	Usually 2 doses	SC or IM	2–8°C	Hypersensitivity to the active substances	After 1 month of the last dose	Fever, local swelling and pain and GI upset	Very rarely any serious reaction is reported, recently included in UIP
16.	Yellow fever	Live attenuated, 17 D 204 strain	All age group >9 months	0.5 ml	Single	Subcutaneous (preferably) or IM	Hypersensitivity to the active substances	Lifelong	Local reaction like pain and swelling, influenza like symptoms, headache	Severe reaction may lead to organ failure, encephalitis and it should not be given with along with cholera vaccine

Bibliography/Further Reading

1. IAP Guidebook on Immunization 2013–14, Indian Academy of Pediatrics, National Publication House, Gwalior.
2. K. Park. Park's Textbook of Preventive and Social Medicine. 23rd Edition, 2015. Banarsidas Bhanot Publishers, Jabalpur.
3. Lozano R, Naghavi M, Foreman K, et al. Global and regional mortality from 235 causes of death for 20 age groups in 1990 and 2010: a systematic analysis for the Global Burden of Disease Study 2010. The Lancet 2012;380:2095–128.
4. National Guidelines on Rabies Prophylaxis, 2013, National Centre for Disease Control, Directorate General of Health Services, Ministry of Health and Family Welfare, Government of India.
5. Roland Estrada et al. Field trial with oral vaccination of dogs against rabies in the Philippines, Biomed Central Infectious Diseases.
6. http://www.cdc.gov/hepatitis/hbv/hbvfaq.htm
7. Sridhar Rao PN. Vaccines. 2006.
8. World Health Organization. Media Centre: Hepatitis B. July 2013. Available at: http://www.who.int/mediacentre/factsheets/fs204/en/

Index

Active immunization 1
Adjuvants 11, 12
AEFI 21, 22
Antibiotics 11, 12
Attenuation 10

Babies need you 41
BCG vaccine 46–49
Boosters 11

Catch up vaccination 14
Chickenpox vaccine 93–97
Cholera vaccine 116–118
Cold boxes 26, 27, 32
Cold chain 23–27
Combination vaccines 6, 15
Conjugate polysaccharide vaccine 4

Deep freezers 25, 32
DNA vaccines 5
DPT vaccine 50–59

False contraindications 13
Fraction vaccines 3
Freeze tag/watch 35

Haemophilus influenzae Type b
    vaccine 104–106
Hepatitis A vaccine 86–88
Hepatitis B vaccine 88–92
Heterologous immunoglobulin 1
Homologous immunoglobulin 1
Hub cutter 20
Human papillomavirus
    vaccine 134–136

Ice lined refrigerator 25, 29, 32
Ice packs 27, 29
Immunization 1

Immunoglobulins 1, 6
Inactivated vaccines 2, 11
Influenza virus vaccine 102, 103

Japanese encephalitis
    vaccine 128, 129

Killed vaccines 2

Live attenuated vaccines 2, 11

Measles vaccine 67–72
Meningococcal meningitis
    vaccine 98–101
Mission Indradhanush 40
Monoclonal antibody 1
Mumps vaccine 75–76

National Immunization Schedule 36, 37
National Teeka Express 39, 40
Needle destroyer 20

Passive immunization 1
Plague vaccine 133
Pneumococcal vaccine 107–109
Poliomyelitis vaccine 77–85
Polyclonal antibody 1
Polyvalent vaccines 6
Preservatives 11, 12
Pure polysaccharide vaccine 4

Rabies vaccine 119–127
Recombinant DNA vaccines 5
Rotavirus vaccine 110, 111
Rubella vaccine 73, 74

Safe injection practices 17–20
Safety boxes 20
Shake test 34, 35
Stabilizers 11, 12

Stem thermometer 30
Subunit vaccines 3
Syringe destroyer 20

Tetanus vaccine 60–66
Toxoids 6
Typhoid vaccine 112–115

Vaccine carrier 27, 28
Vaccine effectiveness 10

Vaccine efficacy 10
Vaccine for travelers 14
Vaccines 1, 10
VVM 33

Walk in cold rooms 24, 31
Walk in freezer 24, 31

Yellow fever vaccine 130

Reader's Notes

Reader's Notes